The Spring Sleep Solution

The Spring Sleep Solution

Matthew Petchinsky

1

The Spring Sleep Solution: Conquering Fatigue After Time Change.

By: Matthew Petchinsky

Disclaimer

The Spring Sleep Solution: Conquering Fatigue After Time Change is a creative, educational, and informational self-help guide designed to support readers in understanding the science, psychology, and lifestyle practices related to sleep, circadian rhythms, and the seasonal time change. The material within this book is intended for general wellness and personal development purposes only. It is *not* a substitute for professional, medical, psychological, or clinical advice, diagnosis, or treatment.

Although this book discusses fatigue, circadian disruption, insomnia-like symptoms, stress responses, sleep strategies, and adjustment techniques, it does not present itself as medical authority. Every human body and sleep pattern is unique. Therefore, the practices, suggestions, and strategies provided are offered as general insights, not individualized medical directives.

Always consult with a qualified healthcare professional—such as a licensed physician, sleep specialist, neurologist, or mental health provider—before making changes to your sleep schedule, exercise habits, supplement intake, medication use, or lifestyle patterns. If you experience persistent insomnia, severe fatigue, sudden changes in energy, breathing issues during sleep, chest discomfort, neurological symptoms, worsening anxiety or depression, episodes of falling asleep uncontrollably, or any other concerning symptoms, you should seek immediate professional medical evaluation.

The author and publisher make no guarantees regarding the accuracy, application, or effectiveness of any strategies outlined in this book. Results may vary significantly from person to person. Your personal outcomes depend on a combination of biological factors, sleep history, environmental conditions, emotional well-being, and consistency of practice. No part of this book should be interpreted as a promise or guarantee of improved sleep, cured fatigue, or permanent circadian stabilization.

The information is presented as-is, with the intention to educate, uplift, and inspire readers to explore healthier sleep habits, increased daytime energy, and better alignment with seasonal time shifts. Any use of the ideas in this book is done at the reader's own discretion and risk. Neither the author, the publisher, nor any associated parties shall be liable for any direct, indirect, incidental, or consequential damages resulting from the application or misuse of the information herein.

This book does not provide medical, financial, legal, psychological, or therapeutic services. Nothing within its pages establishes a professional or clinical relationship between the author and the reader. This work is not intended to diagnose, prevent, cure, or treat any disease or disorder.

By choosing to read and apply the content of **The Spring Sleep Solution: Conquering Fatigue After Time Change**, you acknowledge that you are responsible for your own decisions, your own well-being, and your own health journey. Always prioritize professional guidance when in doubt and listen to your body as you implement any new habits or routines.

Introduction: The Hidden Biological Cost of Losing One Hour

Every spring, millions of people move their clocks forward by just one hour—an adjustment so small it seems harmless, routine, and almost ceremonial. Yet beneath that subtle shift lies a powerful biological disturbance that most people never see coming. Losing a single hour of sleep may appear insignificant, but for the human body, it is the equivalent of pushing an internal system off balance. This book begins with acknowledging a truth few people understand: **the spring time change is not just an inconvenience—it is a physiological stressor that ripples through every level of your biology.**

For many, the disruption is almost instant. Morning alarms feel harsher. Evenings arrive too early to be productive. Brain fog lingers. Energy dips unexpectedly. Mood becomes fragile. These reactions are not weaknesses; they are **predictable neurobiological responses to forced circadian misalignment**. Circadian rhythms—your body's internal clocks—have spent months operating in sync with light cues, meal timing, cortisol cycles, and melatonin release patterns. When the clocks "spring forward," your body doesn't make that adjustment immediately. Instead, it enters a state of temporary confusion that researchers call **circadian jet lag**.

This jet lag creates a hidden layer of **sleep debt**—an accumulation of unmet rest needs that builds when the brain doesn't receive the deep repair cycles it requires. Sleep debt is not simply "feeling tired." It is a tangible biological deficit that affects memory consolidation, immune function, metabolic balance, stress resilience, emotional regulation, and cardiovascular rhythm. Most people assume they can simply "catch up later," but the body doesn't work that way. Sleep debt behaves like a loan with compounding interest: the longer it remains unpaid, the more disruptive it becomes.

Spring time change magnifies this effect because it forces the body to wake one hour earlier *relative to natural light.* At the moment your brain expects darkness, your alarm insists on daylight. This mismatch increases cortisol at the wrong time, delays melatonin release at night, and compresses the window where your nervous system resets itself. As a result, the mind becomes overstimulated, the body remains under-recovered, and the emotional landscape becomes more sensitive. The shift can even elevate inflammation markers, disrupt digestion, and destabilize appetite-regulating hormones like leptin and ghrelin.

Yet very few people talk about this annual biological shock. Society treats the spring time change as a minor inconvenience—something to "power through"—but the truth is that the body experiences it as a real stress event. That is why so many people feel exhausted, irritable, or mentally scattered in the days (and sometimes weeks) after the shift.

And that is exactly why you are here.

This book is your roadmap to reclaiming rest, restoring balance, and regaining energy when the spring shift throws your rhythm off course. Through science-backed strategies, practical routines, and easy-to-implement recovery methods, you will learn how to:

- Reverse sleep debt safely and effectively
- Support your circadian clock during rapid seasonal transitions
- Reduce brain fog, fatigue, and emotional volatility
- Realign your morning and evening cues for natural energy
- Build resilience so future time changes never drain you again

The goal of ***The Spring Sleep Solution*** is simple: to teach you how to navigate the hidden stressor of spring time change with clarity, intention, and biological intelligence. You do not have to stumble through the season. You can adapt quickly, recover fully, and turn the challenge of losing an hour into an opportunity for deeper rest and stronger energy.

Let's begin your reset. Your rhythm is waiting to be reclaimed.

Chapter 1: Why Sleep Suffers in Spring Forward

The moment the clock jumps ahead each spring, the world moves on—but your body does not. Most people underestimate how tightly their biological systems are woven into predictable patterns of light, dark, temperature, and hormonal timing. When the clock shifts, the brain is forced to operate out of alignment with these natural cues, resulting in a disruption far deeper than most realize. Understanding *why* sleep suffers after the spring forward transition is the foundation for repairing it. This chapter uncovers the hidden mechanisms and chain reactions that make a one-hour change feel like a shockwave inside the body.

The Biology of a Forced Clock Shift

Circadian rhythms—your body's internal 24-hour cycles—depend on consistent time anchors. These include sunrise, sunset, meal timing, cortisol peaks, melatonin release, and even temperature changes. When the external clock changes suddenly, your biological clock doesn't instantly follow. Instead, the system responsible for regulating your sleep-wake cycle becomes mistuned.

In the days following spring forward, your brain struggles to match a new schedule that contradicts the timing of natural morning light. At the moment your body expects more rest, your alarm demands activity. That one-hour loss compresses your sleep window and interrupts the slow descent into the deeper stages of sleep your brain needs for restoration. The result is a biological mismatch: the world runs on the new time, but your cells, organs, hormones, and neural circuits still operate on the old one.

Sleep Debt Grows Faster Than People Realize

Most people assume losing an hour is no big deal. But that lost hour of sleep creates **acute sleep debt**, and the biological consequences are immediate. Sleep debt is not a metaphor—it is a physiological deficit that alters your body's ability to function.

Sleep debt leads to:

- Decreased cognitive sharpness
- Reduced emotional stability
- Higher inflammation levels
- Slower metabolic processing
- Lower immune resilience
- Impaired decision-making and impulse control

When spring forward occurs, sleep debt grows quickly because the body not only loses an hour but also struggles to fall asleep at the new desired bedtime. The mind is still calibrated to the old schedule, so melatonin secretion is delayed. Even if you go to bed earlier, your brain may resist. This means many people lose more sleep than the single hour listed on the clock.

Light Exposure Is Suddenly Out of Sync

Sunlight is the master regulator of your circadian rhythm. It governs when cortisol rises, when melatonin falls, and when your body feels alert or drowsy. After the time change, your exposure to natural morning light is reduced for several days or even weeks, depending on your region. This matters more than most people think.

When you wake up while it is still dark or dim outside, your brain does not receive the signal that it's time to be fully awake. Cortisol remains lower than it should be, slowing your alertness, reaction time, and mental clarity. Meanwhile, because the evenings feel brighter for longer, your brain delays melatonin release, causing you to feel wired at night instead of sleepy.

This dual disruption—lower morning alertness and delayed evening wind-down—creates a perfect storm for sleep problems. Your body tries to catch up, but without proper cues, it becomes trapped between biological day and night.

Hormones Enter a Period of Temporary Chaotic Timing

The spring time shift triggers a cascade of hormonal misalignment. Cortisol, the hormone that wakes you, naturally peaks around the time of sunrise. After spring forward, that peak no longer matches your wake time. The body tries to adapt by recalibrating the internal clock, but it takes several days.

Melatonin, the hormone that helps you fall asleep, also becomes delayed. It will not shift immediately just because the clock says it's bedtime. Your brain needs consistent darkness over several nights to adjust.

This hormonal mismatch can create the following effects:

- Difficulty falling asleep
- Difficulty staying asleep
- Feeling tired but wired
- Increased late-night alertness
- Morning grogginess that lingers longer than usual

These disruptions do not reflect a personal flaw—they are natural biological outcomes of artificial time manipulation.

Emotional Sensitivity and Stress Reactivity Rise

Sleep and emotional regulation are deeply interconnected. Even mild sleep loss increases sensitivity to stress, anxiety, irritability, and overwhelm. During spring forward, many people notice that minor frustrations feel larger, emotional volatility increases, and patience runs thinner.

This happens because the amygdala—the brain's emotional alarm center—becomes more reactive when sleep is reduced. Meanwhile, the prefrontal cortex—the region responsible for logic, calmness, and self-control—receives less energy and slower neural activation when sleep debt grows.

The result is a temporary imbalance where emotions feel stronger and rational thinking takes more effort. This is why the week after spring forward often feels heavier, more chaotic, or more overwhelming for many people.

Physical Energy Drops as the Body Struggles to Recover

The spring time change also affects physical energy. When the circadian rhythm is disrupted, the body's repair cycles become scattered. Deep sleep—where muscle recovery, immune repair, and cellular restoration occur—may be shortened or fragmented.

This leads to:

- Feeling fatigued despite a full night in bed
- Slower muscle coordination
- Reduced motivation to exercise
- Higher physical tension
- Increases in aches, soreness, or heaviness

Additionally, metabolic rhythms become unstable. Appetite-regulating hormones (ghrelin and leptin) shift unpredictably, which may increase cravings, fluctuate appetite, or lead to energy crashes after meals. These changes reinforce the cycle of fatigue.

A Small Change Becomes a Multisystem Shock

When viewed in isolation, losing an hour seems trivial. But at the biological level, spring forward is a multisystem stressor. It affects:

- Sleep cycles
- Hormonal timing
- Emotional regulation
- Cognitive performance
- Immune function
- Metabolism
- Energy production

The body eventually adapts, but not instantly—and not without symptoms. Most people push through the fatigue without understanding what their body is truly experiencing. This book gives you the knowledge to work *with* your biology rather than against it.

Spring forward does not have to derail your productivity, mood, or well-being. But to overcome it, you must start by understanding its impact. Now that you know why the disruption feels so powerful, the next chapters will guide you through restoring your rhythm, eliminating sleep debt, and rebuilding your energy with precision and care.

Your recovery begins here.

Journal Prompts

1. **How did my body feel in the first few days after the spring time change?**
   Describe your physical sensations—heaviness, grogginess, appetite shifts, headaches, irritability, or restlessness.
2. **What emotional or mental changes did I notice after losing an hour of sleep?**
   Reflect on mood swings, decreased patience, increased sensitivity, or changes in motivation.
3. **In what ways did my usual sleep schedule get disrupted?**
   Explore when you started falling asleep, how long it took, and how refreshed you felt in the morning.
4. **What signs of sleep debt do I recognize in myself?**
   Consider memory lapses, cravings, slow thinking, or emotional overwhelm.
5. **How does morning light (or lack of it) affect my energy after the spring shift?**
   Write about your mornings—do they feel darker, slower, or more difficult?
6. **What daytime habits made the shift easier or harder for me?**
   Think about caffeine, late-night screens, inconsistent meals, napping, or stress.
7. **What rhythms or routines felt "off" after spring forward?**
   Reflect on changes in appetite, exercise patterns, mood timing, or productivity waves.
8. **How do I typically react when I feel out of sync with my body?**
   Journal about whether you get frustrated, push harder, slow down, or avoid listening.

9. **What have I assumed was "my fault" that might simply be circadian biology at work?**
   Explore where self-blame or misinterpretation played a role.
10. **What would feeling fully aligned with my sleep rhythm actually look like for me?**
   Describe the sensations, mindset, energy, and confidence you'd experience if your internal clock felt balanced again.

Closing Reflection

Spring forward can feel like an invisible thief—stealing an hour from the clock and weeks of stability from your body. But this chapter revealed a deeper truth: your fatigue, fogginess, irritability, and disrupted sleep are not weaknesses or flaws. They are natural, biological responses to an artificial shift your body never asked for. Your circadian rhythm is doing its best to protect you, even when it feels like it's failing.

As you sit with your journal prompts, notice how your answers reveal the story your biology has been trying to tell you: *I am sensitive to rhythm. I am shaped by light. I rely on consistency. I respond to change.* These truths are not limitations—they are maps. When you understand how profoundly connected your well-being is to your internal timing system, you gain the power to work with your body rather than against it.

Let this reflection anchor you:

You are not broken. You are adapting.

And with awareness, compassion, and the step-by-step resets in the next chapters, you will rewrite your rhythm, recover your energy, and reclaim the balance that spring forward temporarily shook.

Your body is ready to realign—and now, so are you.

Chapter 2: Resetting the Body Clock Step by Step

Spring forward may be outside your control—but how your body responds is not. Once you understand why sleep suffers, the next powerful move is to **reset your internal clock on purpose** instead of waiting for it to recover on its own. This chapter walks you through a structured, realistic, and compassionate step-by-step process for helping your brain, hormones, and nervous system realign with the new time.

You are not "bad at adapting." Your body simply needs the right sequence of signals. Think of this chapter as your reset protocol: clear actions, small shifts, and daily anchors that tell your biology, *"This is the new rhythm. You are safe. You can sync here."*

Step One: Assess Where Your Rhythm Actually Is

Before you reset anything, you need to know what you are working with. Many people jump straight into forcing themselves to wake earlier without understanding how delayed their system has become.

Take 2–3 days to quietly **observe**, not judge:

- What time do you *actually* fall asleep (not when you get into bed)?
- What time do you wake without an alarm, if given the chance?
- When do you feel your sharpest mental focus during the day?
- When do you feel your biggest energy crash?
- When does your body naturally begin to feel sleepy—eyes heavy, focus softening, yawning?

These observations show you your *current* internal clock, which may be different from the numbers on your phone.

You can track these patterns in a simple notebook or on your phone:

- Write down "Sleep start (approx)" and "Wake time (approx)" each day.
- Note energy dips (for example: "2:30 p.m.—brain fog, craving sugar/coffee").
- Note any late-night second wind (for example: "9:45 p.m.—suddenly wired again").

This is your **baseline circadian rhythm in real life**, not in theory. You're not trying to be perfect; you're trying to be *accurate*. With that baseline, you can now intentionally move the clock inside your body rather than fighting it blindly.

Step Two: Choose a Stable Wake Time as Your Anchor

Your internal clock does not reset from random changes. It responds most strongly to **consistent cues**, and the most powerful of these is your **wake time**. If your wake time moves all over the place, your circadian rhythm cannot stabilize.

Instead of trying to control everything at once, you will:

Choose one wake time that becomes non-negotiable for the next 10–14 days.

This wake time should be:

- Aligned with your real-world responsibilities (work, school, parenting, etc.).
- Early enough to let you access morning light.
- Realistic—not a fantasy time that will force you into sleep deprivation.

For example, if you *need* to be up by 7:00 a.m., your anchor might be:

- **Wake time anchor: 7:00 a.m. (plus or minus 15 minutes maximum)**

Once you choose this time:

- Set your alarm for that time every day—even on weekends, at least for the first 2 weeks after spring forward.
- Avoid hitting snooze repeatedly; each snooze confuses your system more.
- If you are deeply exhausted, lying in bed and gently waking up with slow breathing and soft stretching is still better than repeatedly dropping in and out of fragmented sleep.

Think of this anchor wake time as the **central pillar** of your reset. Even if your bedtime is a little messy at first, your body will begin to adjust to the stability of waking at the same time daily.

Step Three: Use Morning Light to Pull Your Clock Forward

If wake time is your anchor, **morning light is your engine.** Light entering your eyes in the first 30–60 minutes after waking sends a clear signal to your brain:

"The day has begun. Set the internal clock from here."

To reset your body clock step by step:

1. **Get light as soon as possible after waking.**
   - Aim for at least 10–20 minutes of outdoor light, even if it's cloudy.
   - If you cannot go outside, move near a window and open curtains wide.
2. **Look *toward*, not directly at, the light.**
   - You don't need to stare at the sun; you just need bright ambient light in your visual field.
3. **Combine light with gentle movement.**
   - A short walk, light stretching on the porch, or simply pacing inside near a window can signal to your nervous system that the day is active and safe.
4. **Limit bright screens in the dark before your light exposure.**
   - If your first 20–30 minutes are spent on your phone in darkness, your brain may cling to "night mode" and delay full waking.

Over several days, this consistent morning light tells your circadian system to **shift earlier** and align with the new time.

Step Four: Adjust Bedtime Gradually, Not All at Once

Most people try to fix the spring time change by forcing themselves to go to bed an hour earlier overnight. The mind may agree to this, but the body usually does not. Instead of a single giant jump, use **gradual bedtime shifts**.

You can shift your bedtime in **15–20 minute increments** every night or every other night. For example:

- Night 1–2: Usual bedtime 12:00 a.m. → Aim for 11:45 p.m.
- Night 3–4: 11:45 p.m. → Aim for 11:30 p.m.
- Night 5–6: 11:30 p.m. → Aim for 11:15 p.m.

Continue until your bedtime matches the sleep window you need for your anchor wake time. If you wake at 7:00 a.m. and want 7.5–8 hours of sleep, your target bedtime might be between 10:30 p.m. and 11:00 p.m.

If you are not sleepy at your planned bedtime:

- Dim the lights 60–90 minutes before bed.
- Avoid stimulating conversations, heavy news, or demanding work late at night.
- Reduce screen brightness or use night mode.
- Do a 5–10 minute wind-down ritual such as breathing, journaling, reading a calm book, or a warm shower.

You are **gently nudging** your internal clock, not trying to bully it. The spring time change is already a stressor; your reset method should be the opposite—steady, calm, and kind.

Step Five: Align Daily Cues—Meals, Movement, and Caffeine

Your body clock doesn't only listen to light and sleep. It also listens to **when you eat, move, and consume stimulants.** To reset efficiently, you will bring these daily cues into alignment with your new schedule.

Meals as Time Signals

- Try to eat breakfast within 1–2 hours of your anchor wake time.
- Avoid delaying your first meal so long that your body remains in an "overnight fast" pattern into late morning.
- Keep lunch and dinner roughly consistent from day to day—swinging wildly from 5 p.m. one night to 10 p.m. the next makes it harder to set a stable rhythm.
- Avoid heavy, very late meals close to bedtime, which can spike energy and digestion when the body is supposed to wind down.

Movement as a Reset Tool

- Gentle movement in the morning (stretching, walking, light activity) reinforces, *"This is day."*
- More intense exercise is best earlier in the day or early evening rather than just before bed.
- If possible, pair movement and light: a morning walk is a powerful circadian message.

Caffeine with Boundaries

Caffeine can temporarily hide the symptoms of sleep debt while leaving the underlying problem untouched.

To support your reset:

- Have caffeine earlier in the day, ideally within the first 4–6 hours after waking.
- Avoid caffeine in the late afternoon and evening; after spring forward, your brain is already struggling with delay, and late caffeine adds more confusion.
- Notice if you're using caffeine to override your body's real signals. If your body says "rest," but caffeine says "push through," your sleep debt will deepen.

By moving meals, movement, and caffeine into consistent time slots, you create a **web of signals** that all tell your internal clock the same story: *"Here is when the day begins, here is when it ends."*

Step Six: Design a Simple Evening Wind-Down Routine

To reset your body clock, you must communicate clearly to your nervous system that night really is night—even if your brain feels wired or restless. You do this with a **repeatable wind-down ritual**.

Think in terms of **phases**:

60–90 Minutes Before Bed: Dim & Decompress

- Lower the lighting in your space—lamps instead of overhead lights, screen brightness reduced.
- Switch from stimulating activities (work, intense games, arguments, stressful planning) to calming ones (light reading, stretching, quiet conversation, gentle music).
- If your mind races, jot your thoughts into a "brain dump" notebook so your brain doesn't have to hold everything overnight.

30–45 Minutes Before Bed: Soothing Signals

- Avoid scrolling through stressful content. If you use your phone, keep it dull, soft, and short.
- Engage in a calm cue that your body can learn:
    - A short breathing exercise
    - A warm shower or bath
    - A cup of non-caffeinated herbal tea
    - A simple repeating phrase or affirmation such as, "My day is closing; my body is allowed to rest now."

Final 10–15 Minutes: Transition to Sleep

- Turn off devices.
- Lie down and focus on slow, steady breaths.
- Feel your body sink into the mattress—this is not wasted time; this is your nervous system learning the new pattern.

Repeating this each night anchors the new bedtime in your nervous system, especially in the week or two after spring forward.

Step Seven: Plan for Setbacks and "Off" Days

Resetting your body clock is not a perfectly straight line. There will be nights when you stay up later than planned, mornings when you oversleep, or days when stress hijacks your schedule. This is normal.

What matters most is what you do **after** an off day:

- Return to your anchor wake time as soon as possible.
- Get morning light even if you slept poorly.
- Avoid declaring the whole reset a failure; instead, call it a **detour**.

You are teaching your body over days and weeks, not judging yourself by a single night. Spring forward spins many people off balance—your job is to keep stepping back toward your rhythm, even if progress is imperfect.

Step Eight: Create Your Personal Reset Plan

To make this real, bring it out of your head and onto paper. A body clock reset is easier to follow when it becomes a **clear plan** instead of a vague intention.

You might map it out like this:

- **My anchor wake time:**
- **My ideal bedtime window:**
- **My morning light routine:** (where, when, how long)
- **My morning movement:** (what type, how long)
- **My caffeine cut-off time:**
- **My regular meal times:**
- **My evening wind-down:** (3–5 actions I'll do most nights)
- **My rule for off days:** (for example: "No matter what, I return to my wake time within 1–2 days.")

This book is not asking you to be perfect; it is inviting you to become **consistent enough** that your biology can trust the signals you send it.

Journal Prompts

Use these prompts to turn the ideas in this chapter into insight and action. You do not have to answer them all at once—choose a few per day and return as needed.

1. **Where is my sleep rhythm *really* at right now?**
   Describe your current bedtime, wake time, and energy peaks and crashes as honestly as possible—without judgment.
2. **What have I been blaming myself for that is actually a circadian issue?**
   Reflect on where you've called yourself "lazy" or "unmotivated" when, in reality, your body clock is just misaligned.
3. **What anchor wake time makes the most sense for my real life?**
   Explore options and choose a time that feels both responsible and humane.
4. **What would my ideal morning light ritual look like in my current environment?**
   Consider your neighborhood, access to windows, weather patterns, and daily obligations.
5. **Which habits currently sabotage my bedtime the most?**
   Identify specific triggers—late-night scrolling, stressful conversations, work, sugar, caffeine, etc.
6. **How could I make my evening wind-down feel like a reward instead of a restriction?**
   Describe small soothing rituals that you would genuinely look forward to.
7. **What is one small change I can make to my meal timing to support my body clock?**
   Think about the spacing of breakfast, lunch, and dinner.

8. **How do I usually react when I have an off day—and how do I want to react now?**
   Journal about replacing guilt with a reset mindset.
9. **If my body could speak, what would it tell me it needs during this spring transition?**
   Let your body "talk" about its fatigue, stress, and hopes for rest.
10. **What does a "reset" version of me look and feel like 2–4 weeks from now?**
    Write a detailed snapshot of your energy, mood, and sleep once your body clock is realigned.

Closing Reflection

Resetting your body clock after spring forward is not about perfection; it is about partnership. Your brain, hormones, and nervous system are not your enemies—they are responsive, adaptive systems doing their best with the signals they receive. When you stay up late under bright light, sleep in wildly on weekends, scroll in the dark, and push through exhaustion with caffeine, your body is not failing you; it is simply responding to mixed messages.

This chapter has offered you something powerful: a clear, step-by-step way to send **consistent, compassionate signals** instead. A stable wake time, morning light, gradual bedtime shifts, aligned meals and movement, and a calming evening ritual together create a new map—one that your biology can follow out of confusion and into rhythm.

As you move forward, remember this: every small aligned choice is a vote for your future energy. You do not have to reset everything overnight. You only have to keep nudging your system in the right direction. Spring forward may have taken an hour from your clock, but you are taking your rhythm back—one intentional day at a time.

Chapter 3: Foods & Drinks for Deeper Sleep

After spring forward, your body is not only fighting a clock change—it is also trying to restore biochemical balance. Sleep is not created by willpower alone; it is built from nutrients, hormones, neurotransmitters, and metabolic cycles. What you eat and drink can either support your circadian reset or sabotage it without warning.

This chapter explores the **biology of sleep nutrition**, the **best foods and drinks for deep rest**, and the ones that quietly disrupt recovery. You'll learn how to create a sleep-supportive evening environment through your diet and how to time your intake so your body receives the right signals at the right moments.

How Food Affects Your Sleep Hormones

Your brain relies on several hormones and neurotransmitters to create deep sleep:

- **Melatonin** – your night hormone
- **Serotonin** – a precursor to melatonin that helps regulate mood
- **GABA** – your calming neurotransmitter
- **Tryptophan** – an amino acid used to produce serotonin and melatonin
- **Magnesium** – a mineral that relaxes muscles and the nervous system
- **Glucose** – energy used to stabilize your brain during sleep

If these systems are undernourished, overstimulated, or out of balance, your sleep becomes shallow, fragmented, or delayed.

When the spring time change hits, the body becomes temporarily confused about when to release melatonin and cortisol. Food can serve as a **timing cue** that helps restore order. Eating certain nutrients in the evening can gently encourage your brain to say, *"It's time to wind down."* Eating stimulatory foods at the wrong time can tell your brain the opposite.

The key is not just *what* you eat but *when* you eat it.

Sleep-Promoting Nutrients: What Your Body Needs at Night

Some foods contain natural compounds that signal relaxation, sleepiness, or restoration. These foods are especially important in the days after spring forward, when melatonin and serotonin may be delayed.

Tryptophan-Rich Foods

Tryptophan helps your body produce serotonin and melatonin. Include:

- Turkey and chicken
- Eggs
- Pumpkin seeds
- Tuna and salmon
- Greek yogurt
- Tofu or tempeh

Eating tryptophan alongside a small amount of healthy carbohydrates improves absorption, helping your brain convert it more efficiently into sleep-supportive hormones.

Magnesium-Rich Foods

Magnesium reduces nervous system tension and calms the muscles.

Include:

- Almonds or almond butter
- Spinach
- Avocado
- Bananas
- Dark chocolate (small amounts)
- Pumpkin seeds

Many people become magnesium-depleted during periods of stress or sleep disruption, making these foods invaluable after a schedule change.

Melatonin-Supporting Foods

Some foods contain natural melatonin or stimulate nighttime hormone production.

Include:

- Tart cherries or tart cherry juice
- Walnuts
- Oats
- Milk (contains melatonin precursors and tryptophan)

Tart cherry juice in particular has been shown to increase sleep duration and quality.

Drinks That Encourage Deep Sleep

The right drinks can settle your system gently and naturally.

Herbal Teas

Non-caffeinated teas can help trigger parasympathetic (rest-and-digest) activation.

Recommended:

- Chamomile (contains apigenin, a calming compound)
- Lavender tea (relaxes the nervous system)
- Peppermint (eases tension)
- Lemon balm tea (supports GABA activity)
- Passionflower (enhances sleep quality)

A warm drink also creates a psychological signal of closure to the day.

Mineral Waters or Magnesium Drinks

Electrolyte-rich water or magnesium beverages relax muscles and ease nighttime restlessness.

Choose:

- Magnesium glycinate powder in warm water
- Warm milk or plant milk with magnesium add-ins
- Lightly warmed bone broth for amino acids and minerals

Warm, Non-Sugary Drinks
If you prefer non-tea options:

- Warm water with a splash of lemon
- Warm diluted tart cherry concentrate
- Warm oat milk (rich in natural melatonin)

The temperature, not just the content, signals your brain: *"Night-time is here. Slow down."*

Foods That Disrupt Sleep—Especially After Spring Forward

Some foods interfere with melatonin release, cause blood sugar crashes, or overstimulate digestion.

Caffeine (in any form)

This includes:

- Coffee
- Black tea
- Green tea
- Energy drinks
- Chocolate
- Pre-workout formulas

Caffeine can stay in your system for 8–12 hours. After the time change, your brain is already stressed—late caffeine amplifies the problem.

Sugary or High-Carb Late-Night Snacks

These spike blood sugar before bed and trigger:

- Night wakings
- Sweating
- Heart palpitations
- Morning grogginess
- Increased nighttime urination

Spicy or Acidic Foods

These cause digestive stimulation that keeps your body alert.

Heavy or High-Fat Meals

Large late dinners force your digestive system to stay active rather than shutting down into sleep mode.

Alcohol

It may help you fall asleep, but:

- Reduces REM
- Increases night wakings
- Raises body temperature
- Impairs recovery

After spring forward, alcohol compounds fatigue and delays your sleep cycle even more.

Meal Timing for Circadian Alignment

Your body cares deeply about **when** you eat.
To support your reset:

- Eat dinner **2–3 hours** before bedtime to avoid nighttime blood sugar spikes.
- Avoid late-night snacking unless it's a light, sleep-promoting option (like a banana or handful of nuts).
- Have breakfast within **an hour or two** of waking to signal daytime onset.
- Keep meals at fairly consistent times for at least 10–14 days after spring forward.

Regular meal timing is one of the strongest tools for telling your body what time it "really" is.

Nighttime Snack Ideas That Encourage Sleep

If you need a small evening snack, choose options that support rest:

- Banana with almond butter
- Greek yogurt with a drizzle of honey
- Oatmeal with walnuts
- Cottage cheese with tart cherry concentrate
- Pumpkin seeds and a few dark chocolate pieces
- A small turkey roll-up with whole grain crackers

These nourish your sleep hormones without overstimulating digestion or blood sugar.

Journal Prompts

1. **How did my energy and sleep quality change after eating certain foods this week?**
   Reflect on patterns you've noticed—positive or negative.
2. **What nighttime foods or drinks have consistently made me feel calmer or sleepier?**
   Explore which ones work best for you.
3. **What food habits might be accidentally disrupting my sleep?**
   Think about late caffeine, sugar, heavy dinners, or large evening portions.
4. **Which herbs or teas do I enjoy that could become part of a nightly ritual?**
   List options that feel comforting and sustainable.
5. **How would my sleep improve if I committed to earlier dinners for the next two weeks?**
   Visualize the benefits.
6. **What role does emotional eating play in my evenings, and how does it affect my rest?**
   Be compassionate and honest.
7. **What foods or nutrients do I think my body is craving right now—and why?**
   Tune into your deeper biological needs.
8. **If my body could request one "sleep-supportive" food routine from me, what would it ask for?**
   Let your intuition guide this one.
9. **How can I make my nighttime snack (if needed) both satisfying and sleep-friendly?**
   Brainstorm ideas that work for your lifestyle.
10. **What drink helps me mentally "close the day," and how can I use it more intentionally?**
    Choose a calming evening beverage to ritualize.

Closing Reflection

Food has always been more than fuel—it is communication. Each bite, each sip, each pattern of timing sends messages that shape your circadian rhythm. When spring forward disrupts your internal clock, nutrition becomes not only nourishment but guidance. Your body listens carefully when you provide calming nutrients at night, stabilizing meals throughout the day, and a warm, grounding drink when the world feels too fast.

In this chapter, you learned that sleep is built long before your head hits the pillow. It begins with what you choose to eat and drink; it deepens when your meals align with your natural rhythm; it strengthens when you avoid the silent saboteurs that steal rest from your system. As you move forward, remember that every supportive food choice is an act of realignment—a signal of safety, balance, and night-bound peace.

Let your meals become anchors.
Let your drinks become rituals.
Let your nutrition become the quiet force that brings your sleep back into harmony.

Your body is ready to rest more deeply than ever before—and with intentional nutrition, you will give it everything it needs to do so.

Chapter 4: Tech-Free Night Routines That Work

After the spring time change, your body is already struggling to recalibrate melatonin release, cortisol timing, and nervous-system balance. Technology—especially screens—adds another disruptive layer. Blue light delays your internal clock. Notifications spike adrenaline. Late-night scrolling hijacks cognitive and emotional regulation.

A tech-free night routine is not just a luxury; it is a biological intervention.

By intentionally stepping away from screens, you remove artificial stimulation and allow your body to receive the cues it needs to transition into rest mode. These routines guide your nervous system toward a natural, deep sleep rhythm—something spring forward temporarily steals.

This chapter gives you **four fully designed, practical, soothing tech-free night routines** tailored for different personalities and lifestyles. Each one integrates light cues, sensory regulation, and circadian-friendly activities that prepare the mind and body for restorative sleep.

The Grounding Routine: For the Overstimulated Mind

This routine is perfect if you feel mentally wired, anxious, or overloaded—especially in the days following spring forward when emotional reactivity is heightened.

Step 1: Dim the Atmosphere (60–90 minutes before bed)

Turn off overhead lights. Use floor lamps, salt lamps, or candles (safely). The dim environment signals your brain that melatonin should begin rising.

Step 2: Breathing for Nervous System Reset (5–10 minutes)

Sit comfortably and practice slow nasal breathing:

- Inhale for 4 seconds
- Hold for 1
- Exhale for 6

This activates your parasympathetic system—your "calm down" mode.

Step 3: 10-Minute Physical Release

Choose one:

- Gentle stretching
- Yin yoga poses
- A slow floor-based mobility flow
- Neck, shoulder, and back tension release

When your body softens, your nervous system follows.

Step 4: Comfort Ritual

Make a warm, non-caffeinated drink—herbal tea, warm oat milk, or lemon balm. Hold it with both hands and breathe in the scent. This signals emotional safety.

Step 5: Journal Closure (5–8 minutes)

Write down:

- Three things you accomplished
- Three stressors you are releasing
- One intention for tomorrow

Your mind stops looping when it sees your thoughts on paper.

Step 6: Transition to Darkness

Turn off all non-essential lights. Lie down and feel the weight of the day leaving your muscles.

Why This Works:

This routine closes cognitive loops, reduces stress hormones, calms the amygdala, and increases melatonin naturally.

The Sensory Soothing Routine: For the Body That Won't Unwind

This routine helps if your body feels restless, tense, or unable to settle—even when your mind is tired.

Step 1: Warm Wash or Shower (10–15 minutes)

Warm water relaxes muscle tension and lowers your core body temperature afterward, which improves sleep onset.

Step 2: Slow Self-Massage or Muscle Relaxation

Use lotion, oil, or a warm compress. Target:

- Neck
- Shoulders
- Jaw muscles
- Calves
- Lower back

Release physical stress accumulated from the day.

Step 3: Aromatherapy Environment

Diffuse or lightly apply:

- Lavender
- Chamomile
- Frankincense
- Cedarwood

These scents lower heart rate and calm sensory pathways.

Step 4: Cozy Textures & Weight

Get into pajamas that feel soft, gentle, and soothing. Use a heavier blanket if you enjoy pressure. Weighted blankets or warm quilts help the nervous system release tension.

Step 5: Quiet Resting Ritual

Sit or lie in bed and simply rest. No task. No thinking goal. No productivity pressure. Just awareness:

- Feel your breathing
- Feel the mattress under you
- Feel weight leave your bones

This routine is ideal for people who carry physical stress into the evening.

Why This Works:

Physical relaxation increases GABA activity and reduces internal arousal—perfect for recovering from spring forward fatigue.

The Mindful Wind-Down Routine: For the Overthinker or Nighttime Worrier

If nighttime brings racing thoughts, unfinished tasks, or emotional replay, this routine shifts your mind into neutral.

Step 1: Light Declutter (5 minutes)

Clear a small area:

- Your nightstand
- A table
- One corner

Your brain perceives physical order as internal safety.

Step 2: Guided Self-Reflection (Tech-Free)

Use a printed card, page, or notebook with a simple prompt:

- "What is leaving my mind tonight?"
- "What deserves my energy tomorrow?"
- "What can wait?"

This gives your thoughts a place to land.

Step 3: Mindfulness Walk Around Your Home (3–5 minutes)

Walk slowly, noticing:

- The sounds
- The temperature
- The feeling under your feet

This brings your awareness back into your body instead of your thoughts.

Step 4: Light Meditation (5–10 minutes)
Sit comfortably and try one technique:

- Counting breaths
- Body scan
- Box breathing
- Soft focus meditation

This resets your mental state into calm observation.

Step 5: Read or Listen to Something Gentle (no screens)
Choose:

- A calming physical book
- A printed poem
- A light spiritual or inspirational text
- A gratitude list

You're giving your mind a soft place to settle.

Step 6: Darkness & Release
Turn off lights and allow darkness to signal melatonin release.

Why This Works:
This routine interrupts rumination and allows the mind to shift from analytical to restful awareness.

The Rhythm Rebuild Routine: For People Who Thrive With Structure

This routine is for those who like step-by-step rules, predictable systems, and consistency—excellent for stabilizing circadian rhythms.

Step 1: Same-Time Night Signal

Pick a nightly cue at the *exact* same time:

- A lamp switched off
- A cup of herbal tea
- Putting on sleepwear
- Brushing teeth

This becomes your "circadian ritual bell."

Step 2: 20-Minute Habit Loop

Break it into 3 parts:

1. Physical Reset (5 minutes)

Light stretching, shoulder rolls, or neck rotations.

2. Mental Reset (10 minutes)

Habit options:

- Light reading
- Writing tomorrow's mini-plan
- Gratitude journaling
- Gentle affirmations

3. Emotional Reset (5 minutes)

Deep breathing or a quiet moment alone.

Step 3: 5-Minute Bedroom Preparation

- Dim lights
- Make the bed comfortable
- Adjust pillows
- Remove clutter
- Close curtains

Your environment becomes a sleep cue.

Step 4: Final Ritual

Choose ONE nightly action that signals your brain it is time for sleep:

- A calming phrase
- A cup of warm milk
- A short stretch
- Turning off a bedside lamp

Repeating the same pattern nightly accelerates your circadian reset.

Why This Works:

Routine-driven people respond powerfully to predictable cues, making this ideal for correcting spring forward misalignment.

Journal Prompts

1. **How does my body feel during nights when I disconnect from screens compared to nights when I don't?**
   Describe sensations, tension levels, and ease of falling asleep.
2. **Which part of my current night routine creates the most stimulation or mental noise?**
   Reflect on where technology may be interfering with rest.
3. **Which of the four tech-free routines resonated with me the most—and why?**
   Journal about which one fits your personality or nightly struggles.
4. **What emotional patterns tend to show up for me in the hour before bed?**
   Explore common themes like worry, overstimulation, excitement, restlessness, or avoidance.
5. **What specific cues tell my body it's nighttime—and which cues confuse it?**
   Identify helpful signals and disruptive ones.
6. **What small change can I make tonight that requires no major effort, but shifts me toward tech-free calm?**
   Focus on something doable in 3 minutes or less.
7. **If my bedroom could speak, what would it say about how I treat the space before sleep?**
   Let your environment reveal what's missing or what's working.
8. **What physical sensations tell me I'm transitioning from daytime energy to nighttime energy?**
   Tune into subtle cues your body gives.
9. **How often do I use screens to avoid feelings, boredom, or stress at night—and what could I do instead?**
   Explore your emotional habits around technology.

10. **What would a perfect, peaceful, screen-free night look like for me in detail?**
    Paint a vivid picture—lighting, sounds, scents, timing, rituals.

Closing Thoughts on Tech-Free Nights

When you remove screens from your evenings, you remove the noise, the adrenaline, the artificial brightness, and the emotional whirlwind of constant connection. What remains is peace—something your body desperately needs after the abrupt clock change.

Tech-free routines create:

- Predictable cues
- Lower cortisol
- Higher melatonin
- A calmer emotional baseline
- A smoother descent into deep sleep

Spring forward takes one hour away from you, but a tech-free night routine gives back *so much more*. It restores your relationship to your body's natural rhythms. It reconnects you with stillness. It rebuilds your ability to rest.

In the world of artificial light and constant stimulation, a tech-free routine is not a step backward—it is a step back home.

Chapter 5: Sleep Rituals for Long-Term Energy

Spring forward may disrupt your rhythm temporarily, but long-term energy is built through rituals—small, consistent actions repeated nightly that train your nervous system to rest, reset, and renew. A ritual is not just a habit; it is a biological signal. It tells your brain, *"This is the transition. This is the shift from effort to ease."*

Sleep is not a single event that begins the moment your eyes close. It is a **physiological descent**, influenced by temperature, lighting, emotional safety, hormonal timing, and sensory cues. The right rituals create a predictable pathway into deep rest, and when practiced consistently, they protect your energy long after the spring time change is over.

This chapter gives you **six powerful, repeatable, and research-aligned sleep rituals** that help your body maintain long-term energy, stable mood, and restorative rest no matter the season.

Sleep Ritual 1: The Temperature Shift Ritual

Your core body temperature must drop for sleep to begin. This ritual uses heat and cool contrast to guide your body into ideal sleep thermoregulation.

How It Works

- Take a **warm shower or bath** 60–90 minutes before bed.
- After stepping out, your body releases heat, causing a natural cooling effect.
- This drop in temperature increases melatonin production and signals your brain that nighttime is here.

Optional Enhancements

- Use lavender or chamomile-scented body wash.
- Wrap yourself in a soft towel and sit quietly for 2 minutes.
- Keep your bedroom slightly cool (65–68°F).

Why It Works

This ritual mimics natural sunset cooling and is one of the fastest ways to improve sleep onset.

Sleep Ritual 2: The Pre-Sleep Decompression Hour

This ritual focuses on **mental unwinding**—because even if your body is tired, a busy mind will fight sleep.

How It Works

Set aside a dedicated "decompression hour" before bed where you:

1. **Dim the lights**
   Lower lighting reduces cortisol and increases melatonin.
2. **Switch to low-stimulation activities**
   - Light reading
   - Gentle stretching
   - Queit journaling
   - Preparing clothes for the next day
3. **Avoid problem-solving**
   No finances, no heavy conversations, no "deep thinking."

Why It Works

Your brain transitions from beta waves (active thinking) to alpha and theta waves (pre-sleep calm). This is essential for long-term sleep quality.

Sleep Ritual 3: The Magnesium Wind-Down Drink

Magnesium is one of the most important minerals for sleep, supporting muscle relaxation and GABA activation.

How It Works

Choose one:

- Magnesium glycinate in warm water
- Warm oat milk (naturally high in melatonin)
- Herbal tea with magnesium additives
- Warm tart cherry and magnesium blend

Sip slowly, focusing on warmth and breath.

Why It Works

It calms the nervous system, reduces nighttime restlessness, and supports deeper Stage 3 sleep.

Sleep Ritual 4: The Body Scan Release

If your body holds tension—even subconsciously—it keeps your nervous system alert. This ritual teaches the body to let go.

How It Works

Lying down in bed, mentally scan each body area:

- Forehead → relax
- Jaw → unclench
- Shoulders → drop
- Chest → soften
- Stomach → release
- Legs → loosen
- Feet → rest

Inhale deeply, exhale slowly, and imagine tension melting downward.

Optional Enhancements

- Add a weighted blanket
- Use soft ambient noise (rain sounds, fan hum)
- Pair with slow nasal breathing

Why It Works

The body scan activates parasympathetic nerves and lowers heart rate variability—key for restorative sleep.

Sleep Ritual 5: The Gratitude Closure Ritual

Emotional turbulence is one of the biggest long-term sleep disruptors. Gratitude taps into calm emotional states and rewires nighttime stress loops.

How It Works

Each night, write or mentally note:

- **3 things you are grateful for**
- **1 thing you did well today**
- **1 thing you release until morning**

This gives your mind closure and reduces nighttime overthinking.

Optional

Speak your gratitude aloud for deeper emotional effect.

Why It Works

Gratitude reduces amygdala activation and increases serotonin—both essential for stable energy.

Sleep Ritual 6: The Consistent Cue Ritual

The brain loves repetition. A consistent nightly cue becomes a circadian anchor—something your body learns to associate with sleep.

Choose ONE cue and repeat it nightly:

- Turning off a specific lamp
- Lighting a single candle briefly (then extinguishing it)
- Playing a short piece of calming music
- Putting on a certain pair of pajamas
- A spoken phrase like: *"My day is complete."*

Why It Works

Over time, this cue functions like a conditioned signal—melatonin rises simply because your body recognizes the pattern.

Journal Prompts

1. **What nighttime habits currently drain my long-term energy, even if they feel harmless?**
2. **Which of the six rituals feels the most natural for me to adopt—and why?**
3. **How would my morning energy improve if I committed to just one nightly ritual for 14 days?**
4. **What physical signs tell me that my body craves deeper sleep?**
5. **How does my emotional state shift when I end the day with gratitude instead of stress?**
6. **What nighttime environment helps my nervous system feel safest and most relaxed?**
7. **Which ritual could I easily pair with an existing habit so it becomes automatic?**
8. **What beliefs do I have about sleep that I'm ready to release or rewrite?**
9. **How do I want to feel when I wake up each morning—and what rituals support that feeling?**
10. **If my future self (3 months from now) could speak to me, what sleep advice would it give?**

Closing Reflection

This final chapter marks the beginning—not the end—of your new relationship with sleep. Spring forward may have triggered fatigue, confusion, or emotional heaviness, but your long-term energy is shaped not by the hour you lost, but by the rituals you choose moving forward.

These rituals are more than routines.

They are agreements with your future self.

Each warm drink, each dimmed light, each moment of gratitude whispers to your biology:

You are safe. You can rest. You can restore.

Your circadian rhythm is not fragile—it is responsive. When you provide calm, consistency, and clarity, your internal clock aligns with your intentions. Your mornings grow brighter. Your days more grounded. Your nights more healing.

Let your rituals carry you into the months ahead, long after spring forward is forgotten. Every evening, you have the power to reset, to renew, and to build the kind of energy that lasts.

Your rhythm belongs to you—and now, you know how to protect it.

Appendix A: 14-Day Sleep Recovery Plan

The spring time change creates a shockwave inside your circadian rhythm—but your body is fully capable of recovering when given the right sequence of signals. This **14-Day Sleep Recovery Plan** is designed to realign your internal clock, reduce sleep debt, re-establish melatonin timing, and restore your energy through intentional habits, light cues, nutrition, and nightly rituals.

This plan is not about perfection. It is about **consistency** and **gentle course correction**.

Each day builds on the last, helping your body relearn the rhythm it temporarily lost.

How to Use This Plan

- Follow each day's steps as closely as possible.
- If you miss a day, simply return to the next one—no starting over.
- Keep your **anchor wake time** consistent throughout the 14 days.
- Avoid major bedtime swings.
- Pair this plan with any of the rituals introduced in Chapter 5.
- Keep a notebook or journal nearby for nightly reflections.

Think of this plan as a biological reset button—steady, predictable, soothing, and achievable even with a busy life.

DAY 1 — Establish Your Anchor Timing
Goal: Set your wake time and begin consistency.

- Choose a wake time you can stick to for 14 days.
- Set an alarm for that time and avoid snooze.
- Get 10–20 minutes of morning light exposure.
- Go to bed at your natural time; no forcing change yet.

Evening Focus:
Dim lights 60 minutes before bedtime.
Drink a calming tea.

DAY 2 — Begin Gentle Bedtime Adjustment
Goal: Shift your bedtime earlier by 10–15 minutes.

- Wake at your anchor time.
- Do a short morning walk or stretch in light.
- Keep meals consistent today—especially dinner.

Evening Focus:
Adopt one tech-free activity 45 minutes before bed.

DAY 3 — Regulate Blood Sugar for Better Sleep
Goal: Support melatonin timing through nutrition.

- Wake at your anchor time.
- Eat breakfast within 1–2 hours of waking.
- Keep caffeine before noon.
- Add a magnesium-rich food today (spinach, pumpkin seeds, banana).

Evening Focus:
Avoid heavy meals 3 hours before bed.
Use a warm drink ritual.

DAY 4 — Deep Nervous System Reset
Goal: Reduce internal overstimulation.

- Wake consistently.
- Expose yourself to natural light as soon as possible.
- Do a 5-minute grounding practice (breathing, stretching, or slow movement).

Evening Focus:
Try the "Body Scan Release" ritual from Chapter 5.

DAY 5 — Light-Based Realignment
Goal: Strengthen circadian light cues.

- Morning light exposure increased to 15–30 minutes.
- Avoid sunglasses in early light (unless medically required).
- Limit bright screens before noon if possible.

Evening Focus:
Dim lights even earlier—about 90 minutes before bed.
Reduce overhead lighting.

DAY 6 — Create a Night Wind-Down Flow
Goal: Build a predictable pre-sleep sequence.

- Wake time steady.
- Afternoon: do a light walk or stretch.
- Keep caffeine and heavy sugars out of the evening.

Evening Focus:
Choose a 3-step routine:

1. Dim lights
2. Light stretching
3. Reading or journaling

Repeat this nightly moving forward.

DAY 7 — End of Week One: Evaluate Your Rhythm
Goal: Assess progress and refine.

- Wake time stable.
- Review how quickly you fall asleep.
- Review how rested you feel in the morning.
- Adjust your bedtime by 10–15 minutes if needed.

Evening Focus:
Gratitude ritual (3 things you appreciate today).

DAY 8 — Strengthen Melatonin Pathway
Goal: Improve natural hormone timing.

- Wake at anchor time.
- Get direct light exposure.
- Add one melatonin-supportive food:
    - Tart cherry juice
    - Walnuts
    - Oats
    - Milk
- Reduce screen brightness during the day.

Evening Focus:
Take a warm shower 60–90 minutes before bed.

DAY 9 — Sensory Soothing for Deeper Sleep
Goal: Calm the body fully before sleep.

- Add a relaxing sensory input:
    - Lavender
    - Chamomile
    - Cedarwood
    - Soft textures
- Do light movement throughout the day to reduce tension.

Evening Focus:
Try the "Sensory Soothing Routine" from Chapter 4.

DAY 10 — Simplify Mental Load
Goal: Reduce nighttime overthinking.

- Create a small evening to-do list for tomorrow (5 minutes max).
- Offload mental clutter into your journal.
- Avoid dramatic or emotionally stimulating content today.

Evening Focus:
Do a mindfulness walk inside your home for 2–3 minutes.

DAY 11 — Support Sleep Through Food Timing
Goal: Reinforce metabolic cues.

- Eat meals at consistent times.
- Avoid late-night snacking.
- Have a balanced dinner with protein + complex carbs.

Evening Focus:
If hungry, have a light sleep-promoting snack (banana, yogurt, nuts).

DAY 12 — Strengthen Emotional Safety Before Sleep

Goal: Ease emotional tension that affects sleep.

- Practice a 3-minute calming statement or affirmation during the day.
- Engage in low-conflict, low-stress interactions in the evening.

Evening Focus:

Use the Gratitude Closure Ritual from Chapter 5.

DAY 13 — Reinforce Your Most Effective Ritual
Goal: Lock in what works for you.

- Identify which ritual has had the biggest impact.
- Repeat it tonight and slightly extend it.

Evening Focus:
Deepen one ritual:

- More intentional breathing
- Longer stretch
- Longer warm drink moment
- Extended journaling

DAY 14 — Integration Day: Prepare the Long-Term Plan

Goal: Transition from recovery to lifelong maintenance.

- Wake at anchor time.
- Light exposure for at least 20 minutes.
- Review the past two weeks:
    - What helped you fall asleep faster?
    - What improved your mornings?
    - What changed emotionally?
    - What routine felt most supportive?

Evening Focus:

Create your personal **Long-Term Sleep Ritual**, combining 3–5 habits you will maintain.
Celebrate your recovery—even if imperfect.

Final Thoughts

The 14-Day Sleep Recovery Plan is designed to gently synchronize your circadian rhythm through signals your body naturally understands: light, temperature, food, emotion, stillness, and consistency. By following these steps, you are teaching your body to trust nighttime again, reclaiming the hour you lost, and building long-term energy that no seasonal shift can steal.

Your rhythm is not fragile.
Your energy is not gone.
Your sleep is not broken.

It simply needed guidance—and you provided it.

Appendix B: Evening Ritual Cheat Sheet

Your evening routine is your nightly signal to the nervous system: **"The day is ending, safety is here, and sleep can begin."**

This cheat sheet gives you simplified, step-by-step actions you can follow even when you're tired, busy, or mentally overloaded. Use it nightly, especially in the two weeks after spring forward or whenever your sleep rhythm feels disrupted.

The Core 60-Minute Wind-Down Blueprint

(A simple, universal routine for any night)

0–20 Minutes: Transition Phase

- Dim lights or switch to lamps
- Silence notifications and place devices away
- Change into comfortable clothing
- Do 5 minutes of light stretching, slow breathing, or gentle movement

Goal: Shift from stimulation → calm.

20–40 Minutes: Body & Mind Downshift

Choose one or two:

- Warm drink (chamomile, lemon balm, warm oat milk, magnesium drink)
- Warm shower or face rinse with warm water
- Aromatherapy (lavender, cedarwood, chamomile, frankincense)
- Light reading or journaling
- Gentle self-massage for shoulders, jaw, or neck

Goal: Lower body tension + engage parasympathetic nervous system.

40–60 Minutes: Pre-Sleep Ritual

Pick any one ritual you enjoy:

- Body scan release
- Gratitude closure ritual
- Mindfulness walk around your home
- Write tomorrow's "top 3" tasks
- Listening to soft ambient sounds (no lyrics, no screens)
- Lying in bed and focusing on slow nasal breathing

Finish by turning off the last light.

Goal: Activate melatonin & emotional closure.

Quick Ritual Options (For Exhausting Days)
When you're drained, choose **one** of the three:

1. The 5-Minute Reset

- Dim lights
- Drink warm water or tea
- Sit with hand on chest and breathe slowly for 30 seconds
- Get into bed

2. The 3-Item Closure
Write down:

- One thing I did well
- One thing I'm letting go of
- One thing I'll handle tomorrow

3. The Tension Drop

- Drop shoulders
- Unclench jaw
- Relax tongue away from the roof of your mouth

Even a micro-routine calms the amygdala.

Light Management Cheat Sheet

Light is the #1 signal for sleep timing.
Use this simple system:

Evening Light Rules

- **90 minutes before bed:** Turn off overhead lights
- **60 minutes:** Switch to warm, dim lights
- **30 minutes:** Lamps only (lowest brightness)
- **15 minutes:** Only bedside lamp or no lights
- **Final step:** Total darkness

Avoiding Light Mistakes

- Never stand under bright LEDs at night
- Avoid bathroom lights—use nightlights instead
- Reduce screen brightness early

Light choices = melatonin control.

Sensory Soothing Menu
Choose **1–3** depending on your mood:

Touch

- Soft blanket
- Weighted blanket
- Warm socks
- Neck heating wrap

Scent

- Lavender
- Vanilla
- Chamomile
- Sandalwood
- Cedarwood

Sound

- Rain
- White noise
- Deep hum
- Quiet fan
- Crackling fire sounds

Temperature

- Warm shower → cool bedroom
- Cool pillowcase
- Ventilate the room for fresh air

These cues quiet the limbic system and prepare for deeper sleep.

Foods & Drinks for Nighttime Calm (Fast List)
Choose one tonight:

Sleep-Supportive Drinks

- Chamomile tea
- Lemon balm tea
- Warm oat milk
- Warm diluted tart cherry juice
- Magnesium drink

Light Night Snacks

- Banana + almond butter
- Greek yogurt + honey
- Oatmeal + walnuts
- Cottage cheese + tart cherry concentrate
- Small turkey roll-up

Avoid: sugar, caffeine, heavy meals, spicy foods, and alcohol.

The Tech-Free Night Cycle
Milliseconds matter. Here's your sequence:

Step 1 — 60 Minutes Before Bed

- Put your phone across the room
- Turn on Do Not Disturb
- Shut off notifications
- Switch to analog activities

Step 2 — 30 Minutes Before Bed

- Zero screens
- Soft lighting
- Start winding down physically

Step 3 — 10 Minutes Before Bed

- Breathing
- Body scan
- Silence
- Rest

Tech-free = melatonin "green light."

Emotional Safety Checklist

Emotional friction blocks sleep. Use this quick list:

Ask Yourself:

- Did I resolve or release emotional tension today?
- Did I close out major mental loops?
- Do I need 3 minutes to journal something out?
- Is there anything I'm holding onto that can wait until tomorrow?
- Am I carrying someone else's stress?

If yes:

Do a 60-second release:

"I release what cannot be solved tonight. My rest matters."

Emotional safety = nervous system permission to sleep.

Nighttime Ritual Templates (Plug & Play)

Use these templates to build your routine quickly.

Template A: The Minimalist Ritual (10 Minutes)

- Dim lights
- Drink warm tea
- Stretch for 60–90 seconds
- Write 3 gratitude notes
- Lie down and breathe slowly

Template B: The Sensory Cocoon (20 Minutes)

- Warm shower
- Apply calming lotion or oil
- Use lavender diffuser
- Cozy pajamas + weighted blanket
- Body scan in bed

Template C: The Mind Stillness Routine (15 Minutes)

- Turn off all screens
- Do a 5-minute breathing exercise
- Journal intrusive thoughts
- Read something calming
- Dim lights to near-darkness

Template D: The Full Wind-Down Ritual (30–45 Minutes)

- Light declutter
- Warm drink
- Gentle stretching or yoga
- Evening reflection or journaling
- Body scan + gratitude closure
- Complete darkness

This one creates long-term circadian stability.

Nighttime Don’ts Cheat Sheet
Avoid these 90 minutes before bed:

- Social media
- Heavy meals
- Bright screens
- Arguments
- Overthinking/rumination
- Work emails
- News
- Caffeine
- Sugar
- High-adrenaline entertainment
- Intense exercise

These cues signal “daytime” and block melatonin.

Your Personalized Evening Ritual Builder

Choose **one** from each category to create your custom routine:

1. Light Cue

- Dim lights
- Turn off overheads
- Only lamps

2. Body Cue

- Stretching
- Warm shower
- Healing touch (massage, self-massage)
- Weighted blanket

3. Mind Cue

- Reading
- Journaling
- Gratitude statements
- Breathing exercise

4. Emotional Cue

- Release statement
- Soft music
- Aromatherapy
- Quiet reflection

5. Final Cue

- Turn off last lamp
- Say a calming phrase
- Place hand over heart
- Slow, long breaths

Put these together → your nightly "sleep trigger pattern."

Final Reminder: Your Body Responds to Repetition

You do not need a perfect night routine.
You need a *predictable* one.

Your brain learns through repetition.
Your nervous system calms through familiarity.
Your hormones regulate through consistency.

Even one or two cues repeated nightly can shift your internal clock back into alignment after spring forward.

When your nights become steady, your energy becomes limitless.

Message from the Author:

I hope you enjoyed this book, I love astrology and knew there was not a book such as this out on the shelf. I love metaphysical items as well. Please check out my other books:

-Life of Government Benefits

-My life of Hell

-My life with Hydrocephalus

-Red Sky

-World Domination:Woman's rule

-World Domination:Woman's Rule 2: The War

-Life and Banishment of Apophis: book 1

-The Kidney Friendly Diet

-The Ultimate Hemp Cookbook

-Creating a Dispensary(legally)

-Cleanliness throughout life: the importance of showering from childhood to adulthood.

-Strong Roots: The Risks of Overcoddling children

-Hemp Horoscopes: Cosmic Insights and Earthly Healing

- Celestial Hemp Navigating the Zodiac: Through the Green Cosmos

-Astrological Hemp: Aligning The Stars with Earth's Ancient Herb

-The Astrological Guide to Hemp: Stars, Signs, and Sacred Leaves

-Green Growth: Innovative Marketing Strategies for your Hemp Products and Dispensary

-Cosmic Cannabis

-Astrological Munchies

-Henry The Hemp

-Zodiacal Roots: The Astrological Soul Of Hemp

- **Green Constellations: Intersection of Hemp and Zodiac**

-Hemp in The Houses: An astrological Adventure Through The Cannabis Galaxy

-Galactic Ganja Guide
Heavenly Hemp
Zodiac Leaves
Doctor Who Astrology
Cannastrology
Stellar Satvias and Cosmic Indicas
Celestial Cannabis: A Zodiac Journey
AstroHerbology: The Sky and The Soil: Volume 1
AstroHerbology:Celestial Cannabis:Volume 2
Cosmic Cannabis Cultivation
The Starry Guide to Herbal Harmony: Volume 1
The Starry Guide to Herbal Harmony: Cannabis Universe: Volume 2
Yugioh Astrology: Astrological Guide to Deck, Duels and more
Nightmare Mansion: Echoes of The Abyss
Nightmare Mansion 2: Legacy of Shadows
Nightmare Mansion 3: Shadows of the Forgotten
Nightmare Mansion 4: Echoes of the Damned
The Life and Banishment of Apophis: Book 2
Nightmare Mansion: Halls of Despair
Healing with Herb: Cannabis and Hydrocephalus
Planetary Pot: Aligning with Astrological Herbs: Volume 1
Fast Track to Freedom: 30 Days to Financial Independence Using AI, Assets, and Agile Hustles
Cosmic Hemp Pathways
How to Become Financially Free in 30 Days: 10,000 Paths to Prosperity
Zodiacal Herbage: Astrological Insights: Volume 1
Nightmare Mansion: Whispers in the Walls
The Daleks Invade Atlantis
Henry the hemp and Hydrocephalus

10X The Kidney Friendly Diet

Cannabis Universe: Adult coloring book

Hemp Astrology: The Healing Power of the Stars

Zodiacal Herbage: Astrological Insights: Cannabis Universe: Volume 2

Planetary Pot: Aligning with Astrological Herbs: Cannabis Universes: Volume 2

Doctor Who: Convergence Protocol – The Replicator War

Nightmare Mansion: Curse of the Blood Moon

The Celestial Stoner: A Guide to the Zodiac

Cosmic Pleasures: Sex Toy Astrology for Every Sign

Hydrocephalus Astrology: Navigating the Stars and Healing Waters

Lapis and the Mischievous Chocolate Bar

Celestial Positions: Sexual Astrology for Every Sign

Apophis's Shadow Work Journal: **:** A Journey of Self-Discovery and Healing

Kinky Cosmos: Sexual Kink Astrology for Every Sign

Digital Cosmos: The Astrological Digimon Compendium

Stellar Seeds: The Cosmic Guide to Growing with Astrology

Apophis's Daily Gratitude Journal

Cat Astrology: Feline Mysteries of the Cosmos

The Cosmic Kama Sutra: An Astrological Guide to Sexual Positions

Unleash Your Potential: A Guided Journal Powered by AI Insights

Whispers of the Enchanted Grove

Cosmic Pleasures: An Astrological Guide to Sexual Kinks

369, 12 Manifestation Journal

Whisper of the nocturne journal(blank journal for writing or drawing)

The Boogey Book

Locked In Reflection: A Chastity Journey Through Locktober

Generating Wealth Quickly:How to Generate $100,000 in 24 Hours

Star Magic: Harness the Power of the Universe

The Flatulence Chronicles: A Fart Journal for Self-Discovery

The Doctor and The Death Moth

Seize the Day: A Personal Seizure Tracking Journal

The Ultimate Boogeyman Safari: A Journey into the Boogie World and Beyond

Whispers of Samhain: 1,000 Spells of Love, Luck, and Lunar Magic: Samhain Spell Book

Apophis's guides:Witch's Spellbook Crafting Guide for Halloween

Frost & Flame: The Enchanted Yule Grimoire of 1000 Winter Spells

The Ultimate Boogey Goo Guide & Spooky Activities for Halloween Fun

Harmony of the Scales: A Libra's Spellcraft for Balance and Beauty

The Enchanted Advent: 36 Days of Christmas Wonders

Nightmare Mansion: The Labyrinth of Screams

Harvest of Enchantment: 1,000 Spells of Gratitude, Love, and Fortune for Thanksgiving

The Boogey Chronicles: A Journal of Nightly Encounters and Shadowy Secrets

The 12 Days of Financial Freedom: A Step-by-Step Christmas Countdown to Transform Your Finances

Sigil of the Eternal Spiral Blank Journal

A Christmas Feast: Timeless Recipes for Every Meal

Holiday Stress-Free Solutions: A Survival Guide to Thriving During the Festive Season

Yu-Gi-Oh! Holiday Gifting Mastery: The Ultimate Guide for Fans and Newcomers Alike

Holiday Harmony: A Hydrocephalus Survival Guide for the Festive Season

Celestial Craft: The Witch's Almanac for 2025 – A Cosmic Guide to Manifestations, Moons, and Mystical Events

Doctor Who: The Toymaker's Winter Wonderland

Tulsa King Unveiled: A Thrilling Guide to Stallone's Mafia Masterpiece

Pendulum Craft: A Complete Guide to Crafting and Using Personalized Divination Tools

Nightmare Mansion: Santa's Eternal Eve

Starlight Noel: A Cosmic Journey through Christmas Mysteries

The Dark Architect: Unlocking the Blueprint of Existence

Surviving the Embrace: The Ultimate Guide to Encounters with The Hugging Molly

The Enchanted Codex: Secrets of the Craft for Witches, Wiccans, and Pagans

Harvest of Gratitude: A Complete Thanksgiving Guide

Yuletide Essentials: A Complete Guide to an Authentic and Magical Christmas

Celestial Smokes: A Cosmic Guide to Cigars and Astrology

Living in Balance: A Comprehensive Survival Guide to Thriving with Diabetes Insipidus

Cosmic Symbiosis: The Venom Zodiac Chronicles

The Cursed Paw of Ambition

Cosmic Symbiosis: The Astrological Venom Journal

Celestial Wonders Unfold: A Stargazer's Guide to the Cosmos (2024-2029)

The Ultimate Black Friday Prepper's Guide: Mastering Shopping Strategies and Savings

Cosmic Sales: The Astrological Guide to Black Friday Shopping

Legends of the Corn Mother and Other Harvest Myths

Whispers of the Harvest: The Corn Mother's Journal

The Evergreen Spellbook

The Doctor Meets the Boogeyman

The White Witch of Rose Hall's SpellBook

The Gingerbread Golem's Shadow: A Study in Sweet Darkness

The Gingerbread Golem Codex: An Academic Exploration of Sweet Myths

The Gingerbread Golem Grimoire: Sweet Magicks and Spells for the Festive Witch

The Curse of the Gingerbread Golem

10-minute Christmas Crafts for kids

Christmas Crisis Solutions: The Ultimate Last-Minute Survival Guide

Gingerbread Golem Recipes: Holiday Treats with a Magical Twist

The Infinite Key: Unlocking Mystical Secrets of the Ages

Enchanted Yule: A Wiccan and Pagan Guide to a Magical and Memorable Season

Dinosaurs of Power: Unlocking Ancient Magick

Astro-Dinos: The Cosmic Guide to Prehistoric Wisdom

Gallifrey's Yule Logs: A Festive Doctor Who Cookbook

The Dino Grimoire: Secrets of Prehistoric Magick

The Gift They Never Knew They Needed

The Gingerbread Golem's Culinary Alchemy: Enchanting Recipes for a Sweetly Dark Feast

A Time Lord Christmas: Holiday Adventures with the Doctor

Krampusproofing Your Home: Defensive Strategies for Yule

Silent Frights: A Collection of Christmas Creepypastas to Chill Your Bones

Santa Raptor's Jolly Carnage: A Dino-Claus Christmas Tale

Prehistoric Palettes: A Dino Wicca Coloring Journey

The Christmas Wishkeeper Chronicles

The Starlight Sleigh: A Holiday Journey

Elf Secrets: The True Magic of the North Pole

Candy Cane Conjurations
Cooking with Kids: Recipes Under 20 Minutes
Doctor Who: The TARDIS Confiscation
The Anxiety First Aid Kit: Quick Tools to Calm Your Mind
Frosty Whispers: A Winter's Tale
The Infinite Key: Unlocking the Secrets to Prosperity, Resilience, and Purpose
The Grasping Void: Why You'll Regret This Purchase
Astrology for Busy Bees: Star Signs Simplified
The Instant Focus Formula: Cut Through the Noise
The Secret Language of Colors: Unlocking the Emotional Codes
Sacred Fossil Chronicles: Blank Journal
The Christmas Cottage Miracle
Feeding Frenzy: Graboid-Inspired Recipes
Manifest in Minutes: The Quick Law of Attraction Guide
The Symbiote Chronicles: Doctor Who's Venomous Journey
Think Tiny, Grow Big: The Minimalist Mindset
The Energy Key: Unlocking Limitless Motivation
New Year, New Magic: Manifesting Your Best Year Yet
Unstoppable You: Mastering Confidence in Minutes
Infinite Energy: The Secret to Never Feeling Drained
Lightning Focus: Mastering the Art of Productivity in a Distracted World
Saturnalia Manifestation Magick: A Guide to Unlocking Abundance During the Solstice
Graboids and Garland: The Ultimate Tremors-Themed Christmas Guide
12 Nights of Holiday Magic
The Power of Pause: 60-Second Mindfulness Practices
The Quick Reset: How to Reclaim Your Life After Burnout
The Shadow Eater: A Tale of Despair and Survival
The Micro-Mastery Method: Transform Your Skills in Just Minutes a Day

Reclaiming Time: How to Live More by Doing Less
Chronovore: The Eternal Nexus
The Mind Reset: Unlocking Your Inner Peace in a Chaotic World
Confidence Code: Building Unshakable Self-Belief
Baby the Vampire Terrier
Baby the Vampire Terrier's Christmas Adventure
Celestial Streams: The Content Creator's Astrology Manual
The Wealth Whisperer: Unlocking Abundance with Everyday Actions
The Energy Equation: Maximize Your Output Without Burning Out
The Happiness Algorithm: Science-Backed Steps to Joyful Living
Stress-Free Success: Achieving Goals Without Anxiety
Mindful Wealth: The New Blueprint for Financial Freedom
The Festive Flavors of New Year: A Culinary Celebration
The Master's Gambit: Keys of Eternal Power
Shadowed Secrets: Groundhog Day Mysteries
Beneath the Burrow: Lessons from the Groundhog
Spring's Whispers: The Groundhog's Prediction
The Limitless Mindset: Unlock Your Untapped Potential
The Focus Funnel: How to Cut Through Chaos and Get Results
Bold Moves: Building Courage to Live on Your Terms
The Daily Shift: Simple Practices for Lasting Transformation
The Quarter-Life Reset: Thriving in Your 20s and 30s
The Art of Shadowplay: Building Your Own Personal Myth
The Eternal Loop: Finding Purpose in Repetition
Burrowing Wisdom: Life Lessons from the Groundhog
Shadow Work: A Groundhog Day Perspective
Love in Bloom: 5-Minute Romantic Gestures
The Shadowspell Codex: Secrets of Forbidden Magick
The Burnout Cure: Finding Balance in a Busy World
The Groundhog Prophecy: Unlocking Seasonal Secrets
Nog Tales: The Spirited History of Eggnog

Six More Weeks: Embracing Seasonal Transitions
The Lumivian Chronicles: Fragments of the Fifth Dimension
Money on Your Mind: A Beginner's Guide to Wealth
The Focus Fix: Breaking Through Distraction
January's Spirit Keepers: Mystical Protectors of the Cold
Creativity Unchained: Unlocking Your Wildest Ideas in 2025
Manifestation Mastery: 365 Days to Rewrite Your Reality
The Groundhog's Mirror: Reflecting on Change
The Weeping Angels' Christmas Curse
Burrowed in Time: A Groundhog Day Journey
Heartbeats: Poems to Share with Your Valentine
Dino Wicca: The Sacred Grimoire of Prehistoric Magick
Courage of the Pride: Finding Your Inner Roar
The Lion's Leap: Bold Moves for Big Results
Healthy Hustle: Achieving Without Overworking
Practical Manifesting: Turning Dreams into Reality in 2025
Jurassic Pharaohs: Unlocking the Magick of Ancient Egypt and Dino Wicca
The Happiness Equation: Small Changes for Big Joy
The Confidence Compass: Finding Your Inner Strength
Whispers in the Hollow: Tales of the Forgotten Beasts
Echoes from the Hollow: The Return of Forgotten Beasts
The Hollow Ascendant: The Rise of the Forgotten Beasts
The Relationship Reset: Building Better Connections
Mastering the Morning: How to Win the Day Before 8 AM
The Shadow's Dance: Groundhog Day Symbolism
Cupid's Kitchen: Quick Valentine's Day Recipes
Valentine's Day on a Budget: Love Without Breaking the Bank
Astrocraft: Aligning the Stars in the World of Minecraft
Forecasting Life: Groundhog Day Reflections
Bleeding Hearts: Twisted Tales of Valentine's Terror
Herbal Smoke Revolution: The Ultimate Guide to Nature's Cigarette Alternative

Winter's Wrath: The Complete Survival Blueprint for Extreme Freezes.

The Groundhog's Shadow: A Tale of Seasons

Burrowed Insights: Wisdom from the Groundhog

Sensual Strings: The Art of Erotic Bondage

Whispered Flames: Unlocking the Power of Fire Play

Forgotten Shadows: A Guide to Cryptids Lost to Time

Six Weeks of Secrets: Groundhog Day's Hidden Messages

Shadows and Cycles: Groundhog Day Reflections

The Art of Love Letters: Crafting the Perfect Message

Romantic Getaways at Home: Turning Your Space into Paradise

Purrfect Brews: A Cat Lover's Guide to Coffee and Companionship

The Groundhog's Wisdom: Timeless Lessons for Modern Life

The Shadow Oracle: Groundhog Day as a Predictor

Emerging from the Burrow: A Journey of Renewal

The Language of Love: Learning Your Partner's Love Style

Authorpreneur: The Ultimate Blueprint for Writing, Publishing, and Thriving as an Author

Weathering the Seasons: Groundhog Day Perspectives

Valentine's Day Magic: A Guide to Romantic Rituals

The Shadow Chronicles: Stories of Groundhog Day

Love and Laughter: Fun Games for Valentine's Day

AstroRealty: Unlocking the Stars for Property Success

The Groundhog's Path: A Guide to Seasonal Balance

Groundhog Day Diaries: Reflections in the Shadow

The Groundhog's Light: Illuminating the Path Ahead

Valentine's Traditions from Around the World

AI Wealth Revolution: Unlocking the Trillionaire Mindset

Love Rekindled: Reigniting Passion in Relationships

Single and Thriving: Self-Love on Valentine's Day

Emerald Legends: Mystical Tales of Ireland

Green Alchemy: Harnessing Nature's Magic
The Hearts of Horror: A Valentine's Day Nightmare
The Leprechaun's Guide to Wealth and Wisdom
Dancing with the Sidhe: Celebrating the Otherworld
Shamrocks and Shadows: Mysteries of the Green Isle
Emerald Energy: Harnessing Luck and Growth
The Gingerbread Golem's Valentine: A Sweetheart's Guide to Love and Enchantment
The Celtic Knot: Weaving Life and Destiny
Green Fire: Elemental Magic for St. Patrick's Day
Clover Chronicles: Finding Your Inner Luck
Ireland's Mystical Creatures: A Field Guide
Gingerbread Golem's Love Almanac
Prowl and Thrive: The Lion's Guide to Success
Love Alchemy: Transforming Your Life Through Heart Energy
WORLD DOMINATION: Woman's Rule 3:The New Life
The Midnight Rose: A Guide to Lunar Love Spells
The Forbidden Letters: Writing Your Own Love Prophecy
Luck and Lore: St. Patrick's Day for Modern Mystics
The Green Path: A Pagan Celebration of Renewal
The Dark Architect's Guide to Reprogramming Reality
Prankster's Paradise: A Guide to Harmless Hijinks
Manifest Your Reality: The Law of Attraction Simplified
The TARDIS Owner's Manual: Understanding the Doctor's Ship: *A complete guide to the TARDIS, its technology, secrets, and mysteries*
Starlit Romance: Astrology Secrets for Finding True Love
The Time Lord's Atlas: A Complete Guide to the Whoniverse: ***A breakdown of the locations, planets, and dimensions explored in Doctor Who***
Sweetheart Shadows: The Dark Side of Love and Attraction
February Fire: Reigniting Passion in Every Area of Life

The Self-Love Toolkit: 5 Ways to Embrace Who You Are
February Sparks: Ignite Your Dreams in 28 Days
March to Success: A 31-Day Action Blueprint
Ancient Paths: The 13 Sacred Principles of Dino Wicca
Echoes of Tomorrow: Navigating the AI Revolution
The Wellness Blueprint: Balancing Mind, Body, and Soul
Green Horizons: Sustainable Living for a Better Tomorrow
The AI Wealth Code: How to Make Millions with Automation
AI-Powered Creativity: Writing, Art, and Music for Profit
Extinction Rites: Rebirthing Your Soul Through Prehistoric Magick
Sacred Serpents tarot
Celestial Enchantment blank journal
Star Strains
Culinary Journeys: Exploring Global Flavors at Home
The Hollowvale Curse
The Hollowvale Harvest
The Egg of Transformation: Awakening Your Inner Power
Blooming Into Power: A Wiccan Guide to Spring Awakening
The Nightmare Nexus: The Third Doctor's Perilous Haunting
Digital Detox: Reclaiming Your Life in a Connected World
Ostara's Path: Walking the Spiral of Renewal
The Sacred Hare
Financial Freedom: Building Wealth in the Modern Age
Spring's Cauldron: Stirring the Waters of Change
The Hollowvale Pact
Quantum Consciousness: The Science of Reality Shifting
The Hollowvale Hunger
The Sacred Waters Within: A Witch's Guide to Hydrocephalus Magick
The Raven's Nest: Building a Life of Unshakable Stability
AI and the Human Mind: The Future of Intelligence
The Hollowvale Reckoning

Timeless Love: Building and Maintaining Lasting Relationships

The Raven's Roar: Unlocking Unstoppable Confidence

Raven Sight: Awakening Intuition and Inner Wisdom

The Butterfly Effect: Small Changes, Big Transformations

Taming the Boogeyman: How to Conquer Your Inner Fears

The Magick of Green: Awakening Earth's Energy in You

The Entrepreneurial Mindset: Secrets to Business Success

The Hollowvale End

The Shadow Luck Ritual: Reclaiming Power from Your Dark Side

Spring Magick for Beginners: A Simple Guide to Seasonal Energy Work

Doctor Who: The Hollowvale Conundrum

The March of Miracles: Unlocking Synchronicities in Spring

Unveiling the Cosmos: A Guide to Stargazing and Space Exploration

The Ultimate Guide to Surviving an Economic Collapse

The AI Gold Rush: How to Profit from the AI Revolution

Bastet's Shadow: The Hidden Power of Feline Magick

The Bastet Codex: Unlocking the Goddess's Magickal Secrets

Purring Spells: Harnessing Bastet's Healing Frequencies

Bastet's Nine Lives: Rebirth, Transformation, and Immortality Spells

Primal Currents: Hydrocephalus Magick in the Path of Dino Wicca

The Digital Gold Rush: Mastering E-Commerce and Online Sales

Future Shock: Adapting to the Next Decade of Change

The Quantum Mindset: Think Like a Billionaire

Sacred Motherhood: Awakening the Divine Feminine Within

The Mother's Spellbook: Enchantments for Love, Protection, and Prosperity

The Witch's Guide to Parenting: Raising Empowered and Intuitive Children

The Magick of Motherhood: Reclaiming Your Power Through Rituals

The Pagan Path to Self-Love: A Goddess's Guide to Worth and Confidence

Wild Woman Magick: Unleashing Your Primal Power

The Money Magnet Blueprint: Unlocking Unlimited Wealth

Biohacking 101: Unlock Your Body's Full Potential

The Wild Father: A Pagan Guide to Strength and Wisdom

The Sacred Masculine: Unlocking Your Inner Power

The Druid's Compass

The Warrior's Mindset

The Father's Fire

Odin's Path

Ancestral Bonds

The House That Whispers

The Magician's Code

The Wild Hunt

The Green Man's Path

The Altar of Success

The Shadow and the Sword

The High Priestess's Guide to Energy Healing

The Lunar Mother

The Sacred Self-Care Grimoire

The Womb Wisdom Codex

The Wheel of the Mother

The Witch's Guide to Manifestation

The Q2 Reset

The Ultimate Guide to AI-Powered Passive Income

Escape the 9-5

AI Feline Fortunes

The Tear-Stained Grimoire

Razorblade Runes
Cemetery Sirens
The Midnight Wristwatch
The Town That Forgets
AI Horror & Creepypasta
The Hollow Frequency
The Breach Echo
The Quiet Between Worlds
The Sigil of Tharan-Khul
Summon the Vault of Y'ha'ten
The Becoming Codex
The Profit of Az'ra-nar
The Drowned Logos
Echoes of the Eldritch Will
The Deep Ledger
Necronomicon of Networth
Covenant of the Wealthwyrm
The Whisperer's Manifesto
The Rites of Azh-K'luth
The Ark of the Crawling Coin
The Tithe of Shadows
Inkheart Abyss
The Timewinds of Y'ha-nthlei
The Spiral Labyrinth of Azag-Nirrh
The Gallifreyan Heresy of the Black Pharaoh
The Psalms of Nyog-Sotha
Black Rain Alchemy
The Infinite Maw
The Entropic Blueprint
The Oracle of Sh'guul
The Book of Breach
The Drowned Saint's Testament
Dreamcraft of the Sleeper God

The Silence Market
Cthonomics: The Dark Wealth Algorithm
Invocation of the Ten-Eyed King
Wealthbound to the Wyrm Below
Become the Unnameable
Codex of the Sovereign Flame
Rituals of Relentless Becoming
The Shadow Ascends
The Eyes Beneath You
The Will That Wakes Worlds
Silence Is a Weapon
The Mirror That Screams
The Whisper Between Moments
The Mind That Devours Fear
The Myth of the Finished Self
The Architect of Your Madness
The Voice You've Buried
The Discipline of Madness
Stormborn: Awakening Your Inner Tempest
The Mind That Ate Time
Unbind Your Becoming
The Pact You Owe Yourself
The Devourer's Diet
The Acid That Carves the Path
The Tower You Must Burn
The Breath Between Worlds
Speak Like the Deep
The Labyrinth Within
The Spine of the Sea God
Rejection Is a Portal
The Crown You Refused
The Scar Is the Spell
The Lightless Flame

The Habit of Becoming Horrific
ChickenJockey Chaos
The Gatekeeper Within
You Are Not Your Name
The Compass of the Mad
The Archive of Unsent Letters
What the Mirror Can't Show You
The Knife You Needed
Worship Nothing, Become Everything
The Other Voice
The Body the World Forgot
The Vein of the Void
The Black Bone Codex
The Puzzle of the Hidden Self (Millennium Puzzle)
The Eye That Sees the Lie *(Millennium Eye)*
The Ring of Return (Millennium Ring)
The Rod of Relentless Will ***(Millennium Rod)***
The Tally of the Soul (Millennium Tauk/Necklace)
The Key to the Locked Timeline (Millennium Key)
The Scale of Sacred Decisions (Millennium Scales)
Inferno Bites: The UnOfficial Minecraft Lava Cookbook
Rot in the Attic
Prana: The Hidden Force of Your Infinite Self
The Shadow Realm Within: Transforming Darkness Into Destiny
The Borderland Collapse
Claws of Protection: Bastet's Defensive Magick
Mr. Ring-a-Ding's Madness
Yugioh Astrology: Celestial Deckcraft and Duel Destiny (2026–2027 Edition)
The Seal You Signed: Unlocking the Power You Once Feared
The Puzzle of Infinite Minds: Unlocking the Mentalism Hidden Within

The Eye That Mirrors the All: Secrets of Inner Reflection

Doctor Who: The Toymaker's Broadcast

The Rod of Eternal Flow: Commanding the Currents of Vibration

Golden Eyes of Bastet: Enhancing Psychic Vision

The Key of Dual Forces: Balance Within the Polarity

The Scales of Living Rhythm: Timing the Dance of Life

The Necklace of Hidden Cause: Weaving the Webs of Fate

The Ring of Secret Masters: Rising Through the All Within All

Daggers of the Dying Deep

Bastet's Wealth and Fortune Magick: Prosperity Rituals of the Goddess

The Tide that Speaks

The Scrolls of Petosiris: 13 Rituals from the Feathered Eye

Petosiris and the Living Plague of Osirion

Feline Fire: Bastet's Passion and Love Magick

The Star Altar of Petosiris

Bastet's Whiskers: Supernatural Sensory Magick

The Bastet Grimoire

Feeding the Shadows

The Mouthless Prayer

The Spiral Wound

Becoming the Ibis: Lessons from Petosiris's Mind

The Crimson Coven: Cola Magick for Sweet Dominion

Sacred Cat's Paw

The Soda Zodiac: A Flavor for Every Sign

Covenant of the Crawling Flame

The Ink of Ish'Zur

Frothroot: The Thirst That Ate the World

The Golden Glyphs of Prosperity

The Etherbind Codex

Echoes of the Resistance: Reclaiming the You That Survived

Harnessed Minds: Breaking Free from Mental Control
The Eyes in the Smoke
Rootwake: The Carbon Covenant
Skitter Logic: Unlearning the Fear That Built You
Doctor Who: The World That Froths
Rootwake: The Fizz That Rewrites Flesh
Rootwake: Frothfather of the World
The Holly Pact: Blood Beneath the Mistletoe
The 2nd Mass Principle: Building Unbreakable Tribes
Web of Wits: A Survival Guide to Encounters with Anasi the Spider (Aunt Nancy)
The Hexbreaking Handbook: Effective Spells to Remove Curses
Pop Alchemy: Transform Your Life One Sip at a Time
The Mason Code: Leading in Unleadable Times
Petosiris and the Fifth Chamber of Thoth
The Ether Seed Within
The Parent of Tomorrow
Petosiris's Pyramid of Perpetual Wealth
Unlearn the World
Grimoire of the Hollow Tongue
Zodiac Weeds: Finding Your Strain Through the Stars
Aquarius Rises in the Bank
The Sugar God's Smile
The Skinclock Reversal: Biohacking the Face of Time
Debtburn: How to Obliterate What You Owe Forever
The Ice Cream Oracle: What Your Cone Says About Your Future
Silence Is Sovereignty: The Power of Being Unreadable
The Wind That Whispers Through Stone
Path of the Four Directions
Doctor Who: The Maestro's Symphony of Endings
Oxygen Grail: Breathing to Undo the Clock

Zodiacal Collapse: When Stars Devour Time
Teachings from the Red Sand Silence
Doctor Who: Omega – The Broken Equation
Memory Wipe Your Past: Start Over Like a MiB
Mitochondria Prime: Ignite the Core of Youth
A Nest of Roaches
Grub from the Galaxy: MiB Recipes You'll Never Forget
Whiskers of Power: Bastet's Guide to Inner Sovereignty
The Gift Must Cost Them: Negotiation Through Unequal Exchange
The Worm Guys' Wealth Code: Hustle Like an Alien
Bug Out: The Edgar Method for Ruthless Goal Setting
Weaving Life with Spiderwoman's Pattern
Doctor Who: The Rani's Renaissance
How to Get a Job (If You're a Puppygirl)
Speak Through Others: The Art of Proxy Power
T-Rex Your Trauma: Reclaim the Power of Your Primal Self
The Black Briefcase: How MiB Stay Wealthy in Silence
The Thirst Beyond Reason: Understanding Diabetes Insipidus From the Inside Out
Backwoods Witchcraft for Billionaires: The Pagan Path from Dirt Roads to Gold Roads
The Moonshine Grimoire: Fermented Spells for Abundance
The Nameless Geometry
The Wraith's Mixtape: Spellcasting with Songs of Sorrow
The Gallifreyan Gentleman: Silent Wealth, Sonic Confidence, and the Doctor's Code of Living
Sugar Water Confidence
Dino Totems: Spirit Guides from Earth's First Gods
Pumpkin Sigils & Ritual Smoke
The Hózhó Compass
The Distortus Discipline – Order from Inner Mutation
Witchcraft for the Cold-Blooded Soul

Moonlight Over the Blessingway
Water, Interrupted: When the Body Forgets How to Hold On
Deformed but Divine: Embracing Your Asymmetry
Hexes in the Henhouse: The Farm Witch's Guide to Power
The Reversed Flame: A Grimoire of Inverted Power
Salt, Cells, and Sanity: Reclaiming Balance with Diabetes Insipidus
King of the Broken: Crowning the Flawed Self
Moonlight Scars: Emo Moon Magick and the Art of Lunar Sorrow
Noose Spells: Magick of the Hanging Rope
The Goth Cathedral: Rituals of the Broken and Beautiful
The Cretaceous Codex: Dino Spirits and Fossil Magick
The Turkey Bones Ritual
Nine Lives of Manifestation: Unlocking Bastet's Reality Codes
Chaos Muscles: Building Strength from Twisted Pain
Emo Blood Magick: The Veins of Power
The 3AM Flood: Nighttime Urination, Sleep Loss, and the DI Spiral
The Silence Between the Stars
The Lemon Method: Sour Your Way to Success
Starlit Sovereign
The Rite of Twelve Gates: Walking the Gates of the Duat.
Cornbread and Conjure: Recipes for Riches and Rootwork
The Black Rose Rituals: Emo Love Spells and Obsession Magick
The Eternal Goodbye: Death Magick and Rebirth Rituals
Sinkrot: The Drain That Remembers
The Hybrid Mindset: Thinking Beyond Evolution
Bone Dry: Navigating Dehydration Before It Breaks You
Wreathcraft: Winter Sigils and Yuletide Spells
The Rite of Twelve Mouths

S'mores of the Damned: Haunted Recipes for Halloween Night

Rethink the Drink: A Beverage Survival Guide for DI Warriors

The Shadow Chord: Guitar Magick and Sonic

Malformed Yet Majestic: Leading When You Feel Wrong Inside

The Cursed Diary: Ink-Stained Spells of the Emo Soul

Anxiety Off Switch: Emergency Reset for a Fried Nervous System

The Energy Heist: How to Take Back Your Life from Drainers

Beyond the Bathroom: Rebuilding Your Social Life With DI

Coyote's Gift for Decision Makers

Ghoul-Goo: Spooky S'mores You'll Die For

Echoes in the Mirror: Scrying and Self-Destruction Magick

Thread and Thorn: Stitching Spells from Rural Cloth

The Mogwai Mind: Building Untouchable Wealth from Small Ideas

Be Your Own Guide: Trust Your Inner Compass

Hormones in Chaos: The Endocrine Puzzle of Diabetes Insipidus

ChronoCleanse: Detox Your Biological Timeline

The Limb You Hide Is the One That Saves You

Leaves, Bones, and Whisper Spells

The Dinosaur Mindset: Prehistoric Tactics for Modern Wealth

Clawing Back Control: A Bastet Method for Boundaries and Empowerment

Samhain Codes of the Forgotten

Orange Alchemy: The Autumnal Spellbook

Monster Within, Master Without

The Sigil That Sleeps

Hearthcraft: Yule Hearth Sigils and Winter Warmth Spells

Temple of the Purring Moon: Rituals from Bastet's Lineage
When the Earth Remembers Your Footsteps
Food for Mood: Eat to Heal Depression, Not Just Survive It
Witch of the Kudzu Vine: Southern Pagan Wealth Secrets
The Invisible Diagnosis: Advocating for Yourself With DI
The Coffin's Lullaby: Sleep Magick and Nightmares as Portals
Ashes of the Will: Rituals for Erasing the Self
The Fracture Rite: Shattering the Magickal Core
Funeral Candles: The Art of Emo Flame Magick
The Black Grimoire: A Blank Ritual for Writing in Absence
Phantom Thirst: A Halloween Survival Guide for Diabetes Insipidus
The Hollow Crown: Emo Royalty and Magick of the Outcast King
Sandpainting for the Soul
Falling Into Balance: Using the Extra Hour to Recalibrate Life
100 Southern Superstitions That Still Work
The DI Child: A Parent's Guide to Raising Hydrated, Happy Kids
The Jungle of Shame: Escaping the Hidden Lab of Doubt
The Witch's Toast: S'mores Spells and Creepy Confections
The Hoodoo Pantry: Spells from the Mason Jar
The Immortal Fortune: Secret Wealth Lessons from Captain Jack Harkness
The Specter's Embrace: Magick for Channeling Ghostly Lovers
Grateful Waters: A Thanksgiving Survival Guide for Diabetes Insipidus
The Seizure Gospel
Harvestbind: Autumn Sigils and Samhain Spells
Doctor Who: The Algorithmic Awakening
Silent Nights, Steady Waters: A Christmas Survival Guide for Diabetes Insipidus

The Extra Hour Effect: How One Hour Can Transform Everything

Blade Between the Breaths

Running with the Mountain Shadows

Echoes of the Failed Experiment – Becoming a Living Legacy

Swamp Witches & River Ghosts: Real Southern Hauntings

Cornbread Prophecies: Magical Recipes from a Southern Table

Doctor Who: The Signal in the Star

Bloomcraft: Spring Sigils and Equinox Enchantments

Vanisher: How to Disappear from the Internet Without Losing Your Life

The Ultimate Christmas Cookie Cookbook

The Unbreakable Parent: How to Mentally Survive Raising Kids in a Broken World

Time Debt: How to Reclaim the Hours You Didn't Know You Lost

One Month, One Million: Unconventional Cash Creation Tactics

Doctor Who: The Cyber Conversion Protocol

Black Friday Frenzy: The Art of Finding Hidden Online Deals

The Grimoire Buried Under the Apple Tree

Digital Couponing Masterclass: Your Step-by-Step Guide to Black Friday Savings

The Fire Inside the Flint

Shadows on the Ceiling: The Emo Guide to Astral Magick

The Bone-Eaters Beneath Us

Black Friday Bundle Blueprint: Creating Irresistible Product Packages for Maximum Sales

Thirteen Nights of Unbinding

Doctor Who: Engines of Influence

Pumpkin Spice Alchemy: Recipes of Fire and Frost

When Raptor Met Rexy: Prehistoric Lessons in Wild Romance
Oblivion's Candle: Burn the Path Behind You
Campfire Curses and Chocolate: A Halloween S'mores Grimoire
The Wallet That Wasn't Mine: Breaking Free from Inherited Scarcity
The Cola Zodiac: What Your Fizz Says About Your Fate
Frostfire Fortune: Unlocking Winter's Hidden Prosperity
Signal Jamming: Detox Your Brain from Info Overload
The Dust of the Forgotten Rite
The Golden Cat Sigils: Drawing Power in Bastet's Name
Mud Magick: The Prosperity of Getting Dirty
Savory Spicefall: Beyond the Pumpkin Pie
Pumpkin Spice Apothecary Kitchen
The Pumpkin Spice Economy: Turning Trends into Billions
The Ember Veil: 13 Nights of Fire Magick
Financial Freeze: When Earning Triggers Panic
The Gingerbread Alchemist: Sweet Recipes with a Twist
Biosynth Power: Programming Yourself from Scratch
Echoes from the Talking Circle
Truffle Alchemy: Fungus of Fortune
Spores of Power: The Truffle Witch's Handbook
Doctor Who: The Tower That Speaks
The Mycelium Veil: Truffle Magick Unbound
Broke But Ashamed: Healing the Shame Wound of Debt
The Evergreen Mind: Growth Through Winter Stillness
The Black Veil Truffle Rite
The Voice Beneath Symbols
Witchlight on the Bayou: Swamp Spells for Sovereignty
I Grew Up Poor and Now I Sabotage My Success
The Lantern of Hollow Souls

Shutdown Survival: A Citizen's Guide to Thriving When Government Stops

When Abundance Feels Like a Threat: Healing the Hidden Fears of Enough

The Scarecrow Grimoire

Owls of the October Veil

Candlewax and Curses: A Halloween Spellbook

Excavating the Inner Fossil – Transforming Fossilized Thoughtforms into Tools of Power

The Yule Witch's Spellbook: Magick for the Holiday Season

Haunted Christmas: Ghost Stories for Winter Nights

The Christmas Survival Guide: Thriving Through the Chaos

The Bone Orchard Rites

Haunted Commerce: The Ghost in the Marketplace

When Money Triggers the Inner Child

Silent Night with the Silence: A Christmas Thriller

The Lightning Crown: Living and Leading Through Seizures

TARDIS Tidings: Festive Stories from the Whoniverse

Autumn Reset: Slowing Down Without Falling Behind

The Trillion Dollar Soul: Rewriting the Currency of Reality

Truffle Eclipse Magick

Micro-Manifestations: Quick Magick That Works

5-Minute Rituals for Busy Witches

The Marshmallow Massacre: Halloween Treats with a Sinister Twist

Blood and Blackberry Thorns

Magickal Mornings: Rituals for a Blessed Christmas Day

Embers of the All-Hallows Fire

The Pumpkin Market Collapse

The Hour You Gained: Transforming Time Into Power

The Chamber Must Be Sealed: Mastering the Power of Controlled Access

The Cursed Manuscript of Petosiris

The Festive Hearth: Creating Holiday Traditions

Darkness Rising: Thriving as Nights Grow Longer

Harvesting Time: Turning the Year's End Into Your New Beginning

Petosiris and the 13th Zodiac Key

Wagewound: When Paychecks Become Identity Prisons

Walls That Watch

The Silent Feast: Rituals of Power in the Longest Night

The Distortus Legacy : Becoming a Deformed King in a Perfect World

The Hollow Masks

The Gratitude Furnace: Forging Gold from Thanks

Feast of Inner Gold: Eating for Energy and Enlightenment

Haunted Commerce: The Season of Spending Spirits

Fear Bonds: How Panic Creates Profit

Black Friday E-Commerce Playbook: Sales Tactics to Skyrocket Your Holiday Revenue

Budgeting for Black Friday: A Holiday Savings Planner

Haunting the Harvest Moon

The Warrior's Water: Emergency Preparedness for People With DI

The First Sip of the Year: A New Year's Survival Guide for Diabetes Insipidus

Doctor Who: The Thirteenth Node

The Unseen Struggle: Mental Health, Anxiety, and Chronic Thirst

The Hearth's Hidden Ledger: Counting Energies as Currency

The Gift Alchemist: Turning Any Offering Into Gold

The Papyrus of the Bound Spirit

The Magick of Leftovers: Transmutation in the Fridge

Frost and Fortune: Christmas Wealthcraft for the Modern Magus

Last-Minute Gifts: Creative Ideas on a Budget

10 Secrets to Surviving Holiday Crowds
The Witch's Dow Jones
The Witches' Graveyard Shift
Pumpkin Sigils: Carving Rites for Midnight Power
The Secret Shopper's Black Friday Guide: How to Get Early Access and VIP Deals
Fever in the Foundation
The Neuralyzer Reset: Reprogram Your Morning Routine
Lightning Lessons of the White Painted Woman
The Enchanted Snowflake
The Magic Sip: Surviving Disney Parks with Diabetes Insipidus
The One Who Draws Through You
Santa's Secrets: A Magical Holiday Planner
Silent Bells, Loud Miracles: Self-Help for the Season of Stillness
The Sugar Spell Codex: Confectionary Magick of Christmas
Autumn Hexcraft: Fallen Leaves, Fallen Barriers
Sleep Like a Fortress: Build a Life Where Insomnia Can't Survive
Nowhere Was Ever Home
Christmas Under the Stars: A Celestial Holiday Guide
Rentproof: How to Never Be Evicted Again
Workless: Escape the 9-5 Without Being Broke
The Gilded Gift: A Wealth Altar for Christmas Morning
The Black Friday Grimoire
The Hollowing: Ceremonies of Spiritual Collapse
Doctor Who: The Nameless Signal
Where the Eagle Hides His Courage
The Dwarf Tyrant's Ascent: Claiming Power in a World of Giants
The Currency of the Dead: Trading with Spectral Bankers
The Icebound Witch: Survival and Magick in the Cold

The Emergency Money Mind: Constant Crisis, Zero Calm

Thirst & Roses: A Valentine's Survival Guide for Diabetes Insipidus

Springing Into Clarity: Mastering the Energy Shift of Daylight Saving

Speed of the Nanotyrant: Agile Strategies for Life's Hunt

The 90-Day Reset: A Science-Backed Guide to Reinvent Yourself Before the New Year

The Coil of Thorns

Timegates Unleashed

Dopamine Fasting 2.0: Rewiring Your Brain in a World of Overstimulation

The Nanotyrannus Mutation: Embracing Your Differentiated Form

Unwritten January: How to Use the Blank Page of the Year to Re-Author Your Life

Feast of the Forgotten Spirits: Ancestor Magick for the Holidays

The Burnout Codex: A System for Thriving Beyond Stress

I Don't Deserve to Have Money

When the King Doesn't See You: The Shadow Predator's Guide

The Reset Ritual :A Guide to Shedding Last Year's Weight—Emotional and Physical—by Spring Cleaning Your Soul

Calendar Alchemy: Learn to Bend Time and Productivity around Your Natural Rhythms

The Mirror Contract: A One-Sentence Agreement with Yourself that Unlocks Real Change

The Nile Formula: Sacred Flow for Millionaire Minds

Forward Momentum: Productivity Rituals for the Lost Hour

Harvest Gold: Wealth Magick of Pumpkin Spice Commerce

The Magick of Christmas Lights: Illuminating Holiday Rituals

Cranberry Crown: Royal Self-Worth through Ritual Meals
Petosiris and the Worms of the Feathered Throne
The Evergreen Equation: Self-Help for Sustained Growth
The Rain Will Wash Us Away: Emo Weather Magick
Snowlight Shadows: Magick Under Frozen Stars
Doctor Who: Merger of Empires
The Light Within the Feast: Magickal Wealth of Yuletide Flame
Momentum Machines: Small Habits Designed to Snowball into Unstoppable Forward Motion
Calm Spells: Magickal Solutions for Anxiety Relief
Santa's Final List: The Naughty Never Leave
The Mystic's Guide to Banishing Worry
The Silence Dividend: Turning Quiet Mornings into Compounding Growth All Year
Charmed Stillness: Rituals to Ease the Mind
Blood Spiral Ascension
The Vanishing Heart Invocation
Crystal Calm: Harnessing Stones for Anxiety
The Nano Tyrant Code: Strength in the Small Predator
The Energy Ledger: Accounting Methods for Vitality, Not Just Money
Snowglobe Mindset: Shake Up Your Thoughts, Settle Into Peace
The Weight of the Feather: Anubis's Codes for Soul Balance
Pocket Peppermint Power: Tiny Rituals for Big Holiday Energy
Shadowkeeper of the Golden Jackal: Anubis's Path to Energetic Protection
The Witch's Breath: Anxiety Relief Through Magickal Breathing
The Tiny Ember: Pocket Motivation for Cold Days

Stocking Sorcery: Mini Spells for Holiday Luck and Prosperity

Warm Hands, Steady Heart: Micro Grounding for Winter Anxiety

The Jackal's Lantern: Guide-Lights for Walking the Dark Path

Anubis's Silent Steps: Rituals for Stealth, Peace & Emotional Quiet

The Bonewake Protocol

Extinction-Proof: How to Outlive Trends, Trauma, and Time

The Fourth Doctor: The Eccentric Wanderer

The Second Doctor: Chaos and Charm in the TARDIS (Patrick Troughton, 1966–1969)

The Third Doctor: Earthbound Defender of Time (Jon Pertwee, 1970–1974)

The First Doctor: Genesis of the Time Lord (William Hartnell, 1963–1966)

The Fourth Doctor: The Eccentric Wanderer *(Tom Baker, 1974–1981)*

The Fifth Doctor: Elegance and Empathy (Peter Davison, 1982–1984)

The Sixth Doctor: A Kaleidoscope of Conflict (Colin Baker, 1984–1986)

The Seventh Doctor: The Strategist of Shadows (Sylvester McCoy, 1987–1989)

The Eighth Doctor: A Time Lord's Renaissance (Paul McGann, 1996)

The War Doctor: A Time Lord's Burden (John Hurt, 2013)

The Ninth Doctor: The Healer of Worlds
(Christopher Eccleston, 2005)

The Tenth Doctor: The Lonely Hero (David Tennant, 2005–2010)

The Eleventh Doctor: The Madman in a Box (Matt Smith, 2010–2013)

The Twelfth Doctor: The Rebel with a Cause (Peter Capaldi, 2013–2017)

The Thirteenth Doctor: Breaking the Mold

(Jodie Whittaker, 2017–2022)

The Fourteenth Doctor: A New Beginning (David Tennant, 2022–2023)

The Fifteenth Doctor: Rewriting the Stars

(Ncuti Gatwa, 2023–2025)

Santa's Shortcut to Success: Micro Habits for a Better New Year

The Midnight Cocoa Manifesto: Comfort Rituals for Hard Nights

Why I Can't Save: Trauma Blocks to Financial Planning

Dino Brain, Mega Goals: Rewire Yourself for Savage Success.

Jurassic Profit: Unearth Your Inner Millionaire Fossil

Scales & Softness: Dating with Dino Heart

Carnotaurus Dreams.

Red Willow Thinking.

Reindeer Resilience: How to Keep Going When You're Exhausted

Candlewick Courage: Lighting Strength in Dark Seasons.

Elf-Mode Focus: Fast Attention Fixes for Busy Seasons

Futureproof Feelings: Emotional Skill-Building for Resilience No Matter What the New Year Brings

The 90-Day Rewire: Transform Your Neural Pathways Before Spring Blooms

Jolly Rich: Christmas Micro-Money Magick for Fast Prosperity.

Gingerbread Gratitude: Mini Practices for a Happier Holiday

Trauma-Spending: When Money Becomes a Drug

Goal Skeletons: Build Minimalist Frameworks for Resolutions That Last

The Snarl Strategy: Growling Back at a World That Silenced You

The Hourglass Reset: Reclaiming What the Clock Took

Yule Claw: Dino Rites of Light in the Darkness

Sacred Circles: Grounding Rituals for Anxious Souls

Clockstopper's Gut: Rebuilding the Core of Time

Winterfire Drive: Harness the Cold Season's Stillness to Ignite Deep Motivation

The 5-Minute Productivity Hack: Small Steps to Big Results

Light Ascending: A Self-Help Guide to Longer Days

Inner Economy: Trade Self-Doubt for Confidence Like a High-Value Currency

Simple Success: Decluttering Your Life for Better Results

The Resilient Mind: Thriving in Tough Times

The 2026 Playbook: Mastering the Year Ahead

Get Some Tarot cards: https://www.makeplayingcards.com/sell/apophis-occult-shop

Get some shirts: https://www.bonfire.com/store/apophis-shirt-emporium/

Instagrams:
@apophis_enterprises,
@apophisbookemporium,
@apophisscardshop
Twitter: @apophisenterpr1
Tiktok:@apophisenterprise
Youtube: @sg1fan23477
Hive: @sg1fan23477
CheeLee: @SG1fan23477

Podcast: Apophis Chat Zone: https://open.spotify.com/show/5zXbrCLEV2xzCp8ybrfHsk?si=fb4d4fdbdce44dec

Newsletter: https://apophiss-newsletter-27c897.beehiiv.com/

If you want to support me or see posts of other projects that I have come over to: **buymeacoffee.com/mpetchinskg**

I post there daily several times a day

Get your Dinowicca or Christmas themed digital products, especially Santa Raptor songs and other musics. Here: **https://sg1fan23477.gumroad.com**

Apophis Yuletide Digital has not only digital Christmas items, but it will have all things with Dinowicca as well as other Digital products.

www.ingramcontent.com/pod-product-compliance
Lightning Source LLC
LaVergne TN
LVHW022228200926
848481LV00006B/2176
* 9 7 9 8 2 9 5 4 6 7 6 3 9 *